I0039953

The Doctor in You. © Cesia Estebané, 2023.
All rights reserved. San Juan, Puerto Rico.

ISBN: 978-1-7374235-1-5

Website: www.drcesia.com
Instagram: @drcesiaestebane
Telephone: 787-667-1480 / 787-294-5793

Editor & translator: Yasmín Rodríguez
The Writing Ghost®, Inc.
www.thewritingghost.com

CON TU LIBRO

Emprende Con Tu Libro Self-Publishing Program
Self-publishing mentor: Anita Paniagua
www.emprendecontulibro.net

Cover and interior design: Amanda Jusino
Layout: Anamar Romero
www.amandajusino.com

Photography of the author: Raúl Romero Photography
raulromerophotography@gmail.com

Illustrations inside the book: Anamar Romero
anamartillustration@gmail.com

No part of this book may be reproduced or transmitted in any form or by any medium, electronic or mechanic, including fotocopies, recordings, or any storage or reproduction system, without written license by the author.

All bible quotes are from the *New International Version (NIV), 2011 update.*

This book and all of its content is the result of the knowledge and thoughts of the author. This book does not represent nor claim to be anything other than the sincere opinion of the author about the topics discussed. The purpose of this book is purely informative. While the author and her production team have done everything possible to guarantee that the information in this book is correct at the moment of publishing, they do not assume any responsibility for any loss or damage due to errors or omissions.

DR. CESIA ESTEBANÉ

THE DOCTOR IN YOU

5 Constructs to Discover
Your Innate Power to Heal

I envision a world where humanity lives exactly how they were designed to live, healed and fulfilled in every area.

I envision a world where humanity lives without toxic substances starting from childhood.

I envision a world where humanity carries out our divine purpose according to the desires of every person's heart.

- *Cesia.*

DEDICATION

To you, who are awakening to a new and glorious reality and are on the way to discover the delights of the unknown and everything that is possible, moving away from what is known and common. This is for you.

Table of Contents

Acknowledgments

To my adored life team that share all of my experiences: my family, José, Ian, and Eliam, who always understand and support my passion for writing.

To my inconditional team at any hour or from any distance, no matter what: my parents Martha and Manuel, for always caressing my heart and for the strength from their spirits.

To the guidance and professionalism of Anita, Yasmín, and Amanda in the externalization of this manuscript.

To my most cherished mentors and guides in every stage of my life.

To you, who are in my heart even without knowing you physically: seeing you in my mind and the feeling of connection I have with you are what propelled me to write.

INSIDE THESE PAGES

"The master appears when the student is ready..." That means that Dr. Cesia Estebané, through this book, arrives to you at the perfect moment.

The book you have in your hands may easily change your life for the better.

Inside these pages lie universal truths that govern our very existence. You'll understand more about your mind and your heart, how to liberate yourself from sickness, and how to live a fulfilled and abundant life.

Again and again this book will encourage you to improve, better understand yourself, and heal. It achieves all that through data presented from various scientific studies, which reveal the inmeasurable capacity of the human potential. In addition, it includes practical exercises so you can begin to reconnect with true solutions to challenges in key areas of your life.

Magestically, with ease and elegance, this book reveals the sustained link between quantum energy and the essence of spirituality that characterizes us as human beings. It's written with depth and respect for the innermost part of our body and our being, but also with a simplicity that makes it easy for any reader to grasp.

Dr. Cesia Estebané captured her soul in this literary work, using her faith and compassion to take readers on a mental journey towards what is possible and desired.

Gracefully, she postulates key questions that stimulate critical thinking. She also suggests and explains various mental exercises that open unknown spaces and awaken answers to misteries about our own essence, which then invite us to transcend.

It's a valuable read and necessary for everybody who desires to live a healthy and fulfilled life, in harmony with their environment.

At your service,

Dr. Eddy L. Diaz

LETTER TO THE READER

Dear friend,

Your privilege and inherent birthright is to be completely healed and fulfilled in every area of your life. My goal with this book is to aid you in reclaiming that privilege and right.

I wrote this because I think it's the most appropriate way to communicate the fascinating things I've learned which accentuate and amplify my experiences, health, adventures, and love for life.

As I write, we are living a world-wide crisis. About a year before the COVID-19 pandemic began, a strong craving to write awoke me every night, like a fervent desire to share with you the information I express within these pages. This global crisis further reinforces my intuitive need to communicate this message. I'm confident that this book will fall on your lap at the perfect moment.

I consider myself a lifelong student. The more I study and practice the constructs of life and health, the more I discover the immensity and depth of human potential. Therefore, I now share five constructs that I hope will help to generate health in your life.

To be healthy means to be complete and whole. It is not just being free of symptoms and diseases, but to be in a state of total connection between your body, mind, and spirit[1].

We live at a time where many people are incomplete, living realities that don't align with their lives' true potential. The universe relishes in creation in the same way that you were born to create. You have the innate potential to create a new reality for your life and health.

As a chiropractic doctor, I have had the honor of serving in the healthcare field. I appreciate the privilege of helping others in ways I only imagined in the past that now are a beautiful reality. I've dedicated my last sixteen years to study, live, and share this message with everybody who seeks my help. I've seen how my life has been transformed, along with the environment that surrounds me.

I suggest you read this book slowly, with an open heart and keen mind. Carry out the exercises I recommend as you read and give yourself the opportunity and time to absorb them deeply. This book is my gift of love, and it can be a blessing to you. It reflects my desire to contribute to your quest to live in transcendental health. It can help you be more complete (healthy) and fulfilled, while attracting joy, abundance, satisfaction, and splendor into your life.

May this book strengthen the light that shines within you.

Enjoy!

With love,

Cesia.

CONSTRUCT #1:

Discover the Doctor in You

Your Body's Orchestra

Have you ever listened to a professional symphony orchestra, where every musical detail is of the utmost quality? Do you remember what that experience was like? If it was an excellent ensemble, most likely everything you heard and saw was well coordinated. Every musician had their full attention on the music they produced under the direction of the conductor. You could appreciate each well-tuned and coordinated instrument creating beautiful music that speaks to your soul in a special way.

Your body works that same way. Visualize your body as a musical orchestra, where the conductor is your nervous system and each organ is a musician. Each organ is well-tuned and coordinated with the others, each carrying out their distinct functions under the direction of your nervous system.

For example, look at your heart and lungs working together. Look at your thyroid, your pancreas, and your liver communicating efficiently with each other under the direction of your nervous system. That nervous system is communicating constantly with the rest of the body, guiding and coordinating each function, just as an orchestra conductor guides the musicians.

How pleasant it is to listen to a well-tuned and coordinated orchestra! It can create an enjoyable environment for everyone who listens. The beautiful music an orchestra can generate is equal to the optimal health your body can generate. **Every organ in your body knows its function, just as every musician knows their instrument.**

There's intelligence in every cell, tissue, and organ in your body that always seeks to return to a state of balance and harmony, to its normal state of health. Maybe you have learned that to have good physical health you need to take care of your body, and today I encourage you to think differently.

The secret to optimal health is to allow your body to take care of you.

Modern medicine, with all of its advances, still cannot know what your body knows innately. The doctor is in you. Every single cell in your body has a doctor inside it. The external doctor facilitates your body's healing when something inhibits your body from doing the healing for itself.

Everything you do to take care of your body, like having a constructive perception of your environment and the circumstances you face in your daily life, feeding and hydrating yourself, supplementing, avoiding toxins, and exercising are things you do besides letting your body take care of you.

An example of how your amazing body takes care of you is when a pathogen enters your organism. Your body creates a chain of chemical reactions to neutralize and remove that pathogen from your body. Your body's energy concentrates on your defense system; you have a fleet of immunological cells prepared to take care of you. This is your internal defense system formed by specialized cells.

The immune system is your body's ability to activate homeostasis when facing challenges such as the virus (COVID-19) that we're experiencing worldwide. Your body responds wisely to neutralize the pathogen, you create mucus, to sneeze, and your temperature rises in order to neutralize the pathogen more quickly.

There is innate wisdom in every process of the body. In reality, your nervous and immune systems work so closely that the immune system can be thought of as circulating cells of the nervous system, each of them with an inner wisdom[2].

Have you ever thought about your body's creation? Your father's sperm joined your mother's egg. They formed a zygote, which contains all of your genetic information (DNA) necessary to become a baby. The zygote divides to form a group of cells called a blastocyst, which will become an embryo and later a baby. The cells of the embryo multiply and have specific functions.

All of this occurs quickly in a coordinated and complex way. Around the fifth week of pregnancy, the first organs develop: brain, spinal cord, and heart. Why are these organs the first to develop? Because your nervous system is your body's conductor (just like the orchestra conductor) and it coordinates all the other organ's (musicians) functions in your body.

Today, we know that your heart also has specialized nerve cells. It is truly amazing to see the precision of the human body's creation. Absolutely everything in your body, every detail, has a reason, and every process or reaction is carried out with precision. Your body was created by, and works with, an intelligence of love.

Is it not incredible that even before you were born, everything followed a divine order for your formation? It was a matter of trusting and hoping that your development in your mother's womb would run its course. However, at birth, it seems like human beings are born incomplete, because modern medicine quickly saturates the infant's body with external and toxic substances[3].

As you grow, you continue to believe there is something external to complete or heal you: a new medicine, a novel treatment, always something external. Appreciating your body, being aware of its majesty is the first step to heal and restore. **You create calm in your body just by appreciating it; your cells follow the intention of your consciousness.**

Personally, I believe that there are great changes in humanity's future, especially changes in human consciousness. We will see that consciousness heals more than anything external ever could. This is totally relevant to the current pandemic. The more awareness you bring into your body, the healthier and more resilient your immune system will be, and the more stable your mind and emotions will be. Your body loves it when you pay attention to it; each cell awakens and rejoices. It is a powerful self-healing technique.

Inhabit your body, be conscious of it, because doing this protects you. It's like being at home; appreciate it and experience it in its entirety. Don't just be there out of necessity. The saying "home sweet home" may have another meaning for some through this pandemic, because it is difficult to accept the threat of isolation within their homes for an extended period.

Accepting the present will help you realize that this is a time like no other; you are being given an incredible opportunity to break everyday habits. You can transform your outer home, which is your physical house, but you can also transform your inner home, which is your body. Life happens in the present. Fill every moment of your existence with your absolute consciousness.

Take a few minutes to do this simple but meaningful exercise, which I call "inhabit your body". Read first, and then put it into practice.

Close your eyes, immerse your body in your consciousness. Focus your attention on different parts of your body, starting with your feet, then moving up to your ankles, knees, legs, hips, stomach, chest, arms, hands, neck, face, and head. Feel the life and energy of those parts as vividly as you can. Stay present with each part of your body for a few seconds.

Visualize your body's energy as a wave in the sea that goes from your feet to your head and vice versa. Feel your inner space, your presence in its entirety. Stay with that feeling for a few minutes. You are intensely present in every cell of your body during that time. Do this exercise daily, even when you think you don't have time, because those are the days you need to do it the most.

Your consciousness is the most powerful and healing entity there is.

Your Body's Wisdom and Power

Although you are not just a physical body, it is very important to value and admire that body. There is a constant, innate intelligence that performs various complex functions in your body in an organized way. That innate intelligence is part of your consciousness. The same intelligence holds atoms and molecules in the universe. It is the power that maintains our solar system. It is that innate intelligence that keeps you alive.

You get to experience that power when you live in the present, a truth that many still ignore. It is not just mental; it happens throughout your body. You are that power. I trust that, progressively, this will be more clear to you. Our world is evolving. We are in a stage of change, of revolutionary transformation, expressing our innate and invisible intelligence increasingly. Why do I say that? Because every day there are more people awakening to this reality and because you are awakening to this consciousness. Maybe not everything makes sense yet, but something in you is waking up.

They taught you to find the solution to your needs outside of yourself. However, it is within yourself where you will find what you need. Your health comes from the inside out, not from the outside in. This is one of the most important principles of chiropractic. Every living organism has innate intelligence, an organized and purposeful power. Chiropractic finds and corrects the interferences that prevent that innate intelligence's optimal expression.

I like to explain to children that their body's innate intelligence is like magic that knows exactly what to do inside each of the cells that make up their bodies. Children are the first to accept and believe this truth wholeheartedly. They recognize their innate intelligence more naturally and, in my experience, that is why they can heal faster.

I remember the biblical verse that says that we must be like children to enter the kingdom of heaven (Matthew 18:3); the kingdom of heaven is your internal space, where your Creator dwells, where you connect with your innate intelligence. It is not outside of you; it is in you.

Children are truly amazing. I believe that their most significant qualities are faith, love, dependence, humility and forgiveness. Children have the faith that moves mountains: if mom tells her son that tomorrow she will buy him a cloud, he genuinely believes it. Even if their parents are abusive, they love them. They totally depend on their caregivers for all their needs. They have humility, since they do not know what it is to be boastful. They have a forgiving heart, because they live in the present.

We have so much to learn from our children! That's why they are so often acclaimed by Jesus. To heal, you also have to be like a child and have total faith in the innate power of your body; love your body unconditionally, since there is no greater force; rely on the power that created you; and have a heart full of humility and forgiveness by living in the present. Very few things heal as much as forgiveness.

Your innate intelligence is the power that allows your body to be alive. It is the power to heal, regenerate, adapt, and reproduce. This power never sleeps and does nothing to hurt you. It is the power that turned the breakfast you had today into cells in your pancreas, heart, or liver, to give you an example. It manufactures three million red blood cells every minute, makes your heart beat approximately forty million times a year[4], moves your lungs to use approximately 550 liters of oxygen per day[5], your stomach to produce three to four liters of gastric juice per day, and your nerves to transmit their signals at 268 mph[6].

Your body is truly a wonderful gift - love it, value it, and admire it[7]. Innate intelligence travels through your nervous system, which is your body's conductor. It is your body's communication system.

Sometimes your health may not be ideal, but you can recognize that this is not the permanent state of your body. Your body is constantly changing. You have hundreds of billions of new cells every day waiting to create health within your body. Old cells are constantly being replaced by new cells, and this is how your body maintains homeostasis and health.

Every moment you live differs from the one before. You can listen to the diagnosis the doctor gives you, but do not let your mind linger there. Take the steps to allow your health to restore itself. Your body is truly an admirable gift. It is designed to be healthy with its fifty trillion cells communicating constantly, always changing, renewing and listening under the direction of your nervous system.

Trust in the innate power of your body, because the same power that created your body is the power that can heal it. It is in you.

The Orchestra Director's Helmet and Armor

How important is the conductor of an orchestra? In other words, how important is your nervous system? It is vital. Innate intelligence uses your nervous system to communicate with the rest of the body and thus organize and coordinate its function, healing and recreation. Your nervous system is protected by a unique attire.

Your skull is the helmet that protects your brain, and your spine is the armor that protects your spinal cord. Chiropractic focuses on the conductor of your orchestra and his clothing. It works on the nervous system and its protection, which is your spine.

When the clothing, which is your spine, is in the correct alignment, flexible and moving well, your nervous system can communicate freely with the rest of your body and vice versa, carrying out the functions of healing and regeneration optimally.

Your brain and nervous system are some of the most significant and complex systems in the universe. The nervous and mental impulses that run through your nervous system keep every organ in your body functioning properly, just as electrical cables keep electricity flowing to every area of your home. To have a healthy body, aim to have a healthy nervous system. To have a healthy nervous system, aim to have a healthy spine.

The Unfashionable Orchestra Director

Imagine that the orchestra's conductor is badly dressed. His clothes do not fit him. He is uncomfortable because his shirt buttons are too tight against his chest, his tie does not let him breathe easily, and you can see his clothes are old and even torn. Do you think that amid so much discomfort, he can direct his musicians optimally? It would be very difficult, since he cannot even breathe well.

The musicians then cease to be in sync with each other and get out of tune. Suddenly, you realize that the music they produce as a group is no longer of the best quality. You may even hear noise instead of music, and it is uncomfortable to listen to.

Each musician does what he thinks is right on his own, without a clear direction from his conductor, as there is interference in the communication between the conductor and the musicians. This metaphor may seem strange to you, but I think it can help you better understand how your body works under the direction of your nervous system.

Interference between your brain (conductor) and one of your organs (musicians) is known as a subluxation; this nervous interference causes the organ's cellular tissue to lose its energetic vibration, because communication is interrupted. Subluxation means a condition of less light.

In 1921, medical doctor Henry Winsor was intrigued to see patients heal with chiropractic care without the use of drugs or surgery. He carried out scientific research at the University of Pennsylvania where, in three different studies, he dissected seventy-five human corpses and twenty-two animal corpses. He wanted to look for a relationship between a diseased internal organ and the vertebrae associated with the nerves that reach that organ.

In his results, he found a relationship of almost 100% between the diseased internal organ and the vertebral segment associated with that organ. As you can see in the image, your spine comprises twenty-four vertebrae, which are classified into seven cervical, twelve thoracic, and five lumbar. Each region has a relationship with different organs in your body.

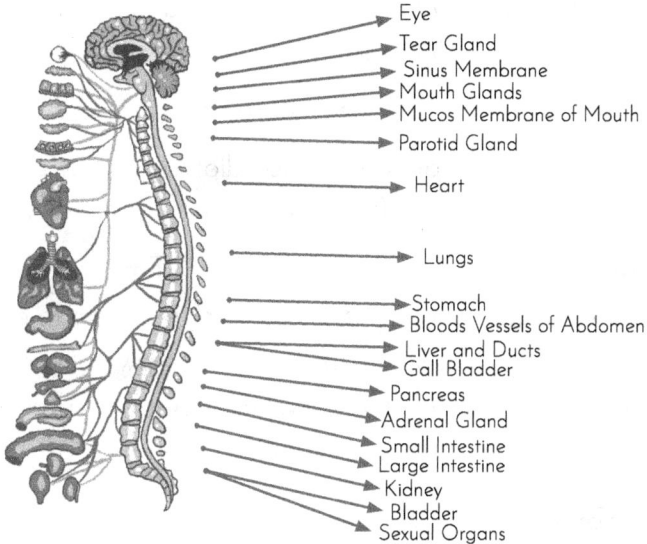

Here are the diseases studied in this research and their association with the spine, by category.

- All nine cases with stomach disease had subluxation in the mid-thoracic area (T5 - T9)

- The twenty-six cases with pulmonary diseases had subluxation in the upper thoracic region.

- All thirteen cases with liver disease had subluxation in the mid-thoracic area.

- All five cases with gallstones had subluxation in the mid-thoracic area.

- All three cases with pancreatic diseases had subluxation in the mid-thoracic area.

- All eleven cases with spleen diseases had subluxation in the mid-thoracic area.

- All seventeen cases with kidney disease had subluxation in the lower thoracic area.

- The eight cases with prostate and bladder diseases had subluxation in the lumbar area (L2-L3).

- The two cases with uterine disease had L2 subluxation.

- The cases with heart and pericardial conditions presented subluxation in the first five thoracic areas (T1-T5).

These results were published in the *Medical Times* and have led to extensive research on the relationship of the spine to each organ. By presenting this study, my goal is to show how important it is to have an optimal nervous system, free of interference, for a better expression of life and health.

Subluxation (interference) is much more than a vertebra out of place: it is a condition of less light, because it interrupts the flow of energy in the body. The chiropractor detects, analyzes, and corrects subluxation to facilitate the flow of energy.

Subluxation (interference) can occur at a very young age, as early as birth, because of the effects of stressors on your body. Understanding these stressors will be of great benefit.

We mainly divide stressors into three categories: emotional stress, chemical stress, and physical stress. Which stressor do you think creates the most damage and subluxation in your body? Without a doubt, it is the emotional stress; you are a spiritual being living a physical life experience. For this reason, your body responds more to emotional stress than to chemical and physical stress.

Chemical stress is the second most demanding stressor in your body. It is caused mainly by chemicals in prescription and non-prescription drugs, vaccines, products for home cleaning or for personal use, preservatives and additives in our food, and pollution in our environment.

Physical stress is the one that represents the least burden on your body. However, it includes the birth process for a newborn. The force exerted to remove the baby's head from the mother's body can place great stress on the baby's spine, and from that day onward, the child may present vertebral subluxations. In addition, repetitive work, incorrect posture habits, falls from an early age, and accidents may also cause them.

Subluxation is part of the law of entropy, which explains that the body becomes disordered, weak and deteriorated under different stressors. The purpose of chiropractic adjustment is to restore the flow of life-giving energy and to always seek syntropy (order) rather than entropy (disorder).

Studies show people who take care of their nervous system with chiropractic care are healthier patients. According to the Journal of Manipulative and Physiologic Therapeutics (JMPT), 311 chiropractic patients, 65 years and older, who received "maintenance care" for five years or more were compared with healthy citizens of the same ages.

The results showed that patients under chiropractic care had 60.2% fewer hospitalizations, 59% fewer hospitalized days, 62% fewer outpatient surgeries, and 85% fewer pharmacy costs. Reversing the law of entropy is possible because your body responds to quantum physics, which recognizes everything as energy, including that which you cannot see.

Taking care of your nervous system is taking care of your body's healing energy. Your healing requires your participation by being aware that your body can repair itself. This is the first step. Chiropractic care, as part of your lifestyle, is an important portion of your repair strategy when different stressors impact your life's timeline, which is reflected in your spine.

Chiropractic and the Musical Composition of Your Life

Chiropractic is an act of genuine **love** for each person who seeks help. It does not treat conditions or diseases; its focus is on **raising the organism's potential to where it can heal itself,** because it recognizes the innate intelligence within each body.

Chiropractic recognizes that the most important doctor is within each person. Its main function is to facilitate the removal of neurological interferences from the body to restore internal communications within the cell and thus maximize the organism's expression of life. It is like removing a veil that obscures the orchestra's conductor; if the musicians can see the conductor clearly, he is more efficient.

People benefit more from chiropractic care when they know its true role. Chiropractic care works under optimal conditions when most patients understand its genuine purpose.

People that do not know the great purpose of chiropractic can limit themselves to think that it is only for relief of symptoms such as headaches, neck pain, and middle back or lower back pain, to name a few. In reality, **chiropractic unites the physical body with the internal doctor by removing interferences in the body and thus allowing it to self-heal.**

Healing comes from the inside. Pain is not the problem; pain is how your body communicates to let you know that you need to pay attention.

Pain is like jarring notes in the performance that the conductor can solve by going to the root of the problem. Pain relief accounts for only 2% of all the abundant benefits of chiropractic care. The body can and will rid itself of symptoms once the root cause is removed.

Chiropractic responds to quantum physics, or the invisible field of information and intelligence; it reconnects the organism with the magnificent spirit within, giving it the potential to heal.

The chiropractor's job is to connect your physical self with your innate intelligence. It is destructive to think that health always depends on something external. Have you ever wondered why, despite having more scientific advances, more technology and more drugs, we have an increasingly sick society?

You are the main composer of your life and health. I hope you recognize the doctor who has always been in you, and that you can heal by trusting that your body is here to support you and is never against you.

Many might think that health can be bought, because money can buy new drugs or medicines to treat different ailments such as heart disease, cancer or autoimmune diseases without getting to the root of the problem. These people have not yet come to recognize that it is their daily actions that contribute to these conditions' high incidence. The more our society grows, the more it depends on drugs to solve everyday problems.

As a society, we are not experiencing good health. The most common diseases reflect our modern way of life. They are lifestyle diseases stemming from low consciousness. Perhaps you have divorced yourself from the responsibility of your own health. The belief that your health depends on the combination of good medications, good doctors, and good hospitals is the driving force in today's healthcare system.

I remember crying on my graduation day because I felt uncertain about the world that awaited me. I felt a lump in my throat that did not let me breathe well but, at the same time, I wanted to show happiness to my family and friends who traveled far to be with me on that important day. The comfort of school, books, and classes brought me there. I understood that school represented security; it was all I'd known.

I had to get out of my comfort zone and move past my fears and limiting thoughts. I recognized it was not just about me, but about many other people. Going into a chiropractic practice was not about acquiring a lot of new machinery or techniques (while there is nothing wrong with that), but being a chiropractor went deeper. I already had what I needed: a clear intention, an open heart, and my hands to carry out my purpose with everyone who sought my help.

Healing your life and your body begins in the inner space of your being. When every area of your life is full of light, you will fill others with that light. There is something very magical and beautiful about acknowledging this truth; whatever your purpose is on this Earth, you already have what you need to heal and carry it out.

Now is the time to recognize and reconnect with the doctor in you. Often, the most common internal battle is between the innermost part that wants healing and the part that is comfortable with what is well known. You are here for a great purpose; we do not serve the world by hiding ourselves, keeping with the regular and comfortable, fearing the unknown and the possible. Recognize that your potential for life and health is not just about you, it is about the many lives that your legacy will impact.

CONSTRUCT #2:

Return to Your Essence

Your Identity - Discover Who You Are

Can you remember your childhood from when you were only four or five years old? Do you remember the way you saw the world? How did you see nature, animals, the sky? How did you see other children? Remember your childhood for a few minutes. You lived in a world of imagination, delight, adventure, and with a sense of wonderment, did you not?

Maybe you have small children, or grandchildren, and you've had experiences like mine. My five- and seven-year-old kids remind me daily of what it's like to live with a feeling of wonderment. They are amazed by every detail of nature and everything that surrounds them. They are attentive to the simple details of a seed, and admire the structure of a little worm. They discover beauty in the rocks they find at random, and that is why I have a large collection of various sizes and colors. Their stories are endless, since their imagination knows no limits. They certainly remind me of the greatness of living with a sense of wonderment.

When you were born, you were a complete and flawless creation. You had a natural inclination to focus on love. Your imagination was creative and cultivated, and you innately knew how to use it. It connected you to a more abundant world. You lived in a world of splendor and with greater sensitivity to the surrounding details.

What changed? Why do magic and fascination fade when you reach a certain age? I will tell you why. You programmed your subconscious, based on what you were taught, to see the world in a way that is opposed to who you are, to think unnaturally. They taught you to have thoughts of criticism, competition, strife, illness, limitations, defeat, failure, lack, and loss. You programmed these things in your mind and that is how you got to know them.

Maybe you learned that doing things the right or almost perfect way is more important than love. Perhaps you learned to seek distance and separation from other people instead of unity, cooperation, and understanding. You learned you had to compete to progress or excel.

Maybe you never realized the innate truth that you are good and loved just the way you are, and you persistently seek recognition from the outside. Perhaps you learned God is the one that punishes, always seeking to judge every sin, and you failed to see or experience his true essence of infinite love for yourself. You are not here to be blamed, punished, or sentenced. If you go back to your essence, you will understand that life is really noble and benign.

Your mind was programmed to perceive your surroundings just the same as others do; the way the world perceives things is not founded on love, but on fear and mistrust.

Your essence, when you arrive on this planet, is love; it is not the fear you have learned since.

That fear comes from not knowing who you really are and not trusting that life is there to support you. Examine whether most of the decisions you have made, and still make, were under the influence of fear or love.

Do you eat healthy and exercise out of love and gratitude to your body or out of fear of getting sick? Do you guide your children because you love them and trust their great potential, or are there internal reasons based on fear and mistrust? For example, you may fear that they will embarrass you or that they will not learn to fend for themselves.

Changing from fear to love is something really significant that affects everything you do. Your essence is the most powerful force that exists. When you decide under the influence of your essence, the effect will be beautiful and fulfilling.

Look at absolutely everything in your world with love and gratitude, and see how it will lead you to places of deep peace, joy, and fulfillment. Get out of your own way, lower the mental noise that fear generates, and show off your greatness.

True Love

As I write this chapter, the month of February begins. Everywhere I look, I see hearts, and the color red is in every store. We know February as the month of love and friendship. However, what I want to convey to you goes beyond what we could consider commercial or superficial love, or some pretty words.

Love is our womb, our essential truth, the reason we are here. The foundation of life is to awaken to this truth, and to experience love in yourself and in others. There is no force more healing or powerful than this.

In order to heal, you need an environment of love, not fear. **Your body can heal as long as you change your perceptions and limiting beliefs.** Your biology changes by changing the way you perceive the outside world. Visualize your body as a large community of fifty trillion cells. Love produces a chemistry in your body that makes your cells grow. The chemistry that fear produces makes your cells protect themselves. Your cells are continually growing or protecting themselves.

When your cells are in a protective state they do not grow, they try to survive as long as possible, but they do not allow growth or regeneration. How would your body respond if some animal was about to attack you? How does your body react to receiving unexpected news that cause anxiety?

At these times, your cells produce stress hormones, such as cortisol, glucagon, and adrenaline. These hormones signal that your body should be in protection mode and then your cells stop growing. The most important thing for your cells at that precise moment is to survive, to protect themselves.

It's natural for your body to respond like this when there's an emergency event; what is not healthy is your body remaining under the influence of stress hormones, merely surviving and protecting itself, for most of your life. Have you ever seen a person who is scared of everything? Did you notice how they shrink, lower their head, enclose and protect themselves, as if they had a shell and wanted to hide in it? Your cells do the same when you are under the influence of fear: they protect themselves to survive.

Think about your daily life and the different stressors to which you expose yourself day and night. How do you respond to them? Imagine this scenario: you get home and your partner argues with you about something. Your kids need help to finish their assignments or finishing studying for a test the next day. At that very moment, your boss sends you a message telling you he needs you earlier in the morning. Your dog begs you to take care of him and you have not even been able to put your things down, or take off your uncomfortable shoes, much less eat dinner. How do you respond? Perhaps because of your desperation, you speak louder than usual to your partner and your children, or perhaps you cry because you feel powerless and frustrated at that moment.

Your response to situations in your life depends on how you perceive them and on your state of consciousness at that moment. If you are living in your essence of love, with consciousness, you can re-frame the "chaos" that presents itself to you. The very presence of love in you will change that charged energy that you found upon entering your home. It is something amazing that you can only understand by experiencing it in your life.

By being in your essence of love, you help others to do the same. Things and people take a miraculous turn, and everything fits and flows. Your story changes.

Imagine arriving home in a state of elevated consciousness and feeling truly connected to your essence. Now you can see beyond the situation presented to you. It is possible to listen to your partner with a peaceful mind and an open heart. You know deep inside that your partner, in the depths of their being, does not really want to argue. You can see the situation with compassion and love. You see yourself in your partner. You put yourself in their shoes and you can understand why they are upset. You listen to them without judging. Keywords emerge within you that help you stay in tune with yourself and elevate your consciousness.

Love is not love until it is unconditional. You do not return the argumentative tone of voice they use; you speak to them with a tone that reflects peace and love. Your words are energy. You do not see them, but they transform your environment. You do not defend yourself, as this places too much importance on trivial matters.

By not trying to be right, you show that your strength comes from within and not from external opinions. You can have peace despite any circumstance. Your partner can be one of the people who helps you grow the most, if you allow it.

Your state of consciousness and energy changes your home environment. You hug your children and remind them how much you love them. You sit with them just to look at them and hug them for a few brief moments. Your partner joins the family embrace, and everything changes from tension to fluidity, from fear to love. Without fail, your pet approaches. It is so intelligent it perceives everything. After those brief minutes of just enjoying their presence, you realize how blessed you are to be alive and together with them. You all realign your priorities at that moment.

This may seem like a bit of an exaggeration because perhaps you are used to allowing your analytical mind to control the situation in other ways, perhaps with a raised tone of voice and fights that do not lead to peace or unity. If you live connected to your true essence, you will understand the power that lies within you. You will see beautiful changes in your daily life.

You are a spiritual being living in this time, and on this planet that fosters so much creation. Allow nothing and no one to take away your power; own who you really are. You are love, a piece of God who came here to create, not with your strength, but with your essence. Your spiritual goal is to let go of fear and accept love back in your life. This is the way back to your essence, to your nature, for there lies your power. Love is in everything around you, every day of your life. Waking up to this reality is like being a fish that always tries to find the sea and finally, one day, realizes that it has been living there since the beginning of time.

All that is essential is within us, and not in the external or material. **To give more value to material things is to love what cannot love you back.** It is the same as looking for meaning in something superficial or insubstantial. Have you ever received a beautiful, even expensive gift, from a person who did not really show love or interest in you, or worse, mistreated you? You can see how the most significant gift is the love that a person can offer.

It is possible to devalue what you know is essential in your heart and overvalue what you only perceive with your physical eyes. One of my favorite phrases is by Antoine de Saint Exupéry: "It is only with the heart that one can see well, what is essential is invisible to our physical sight."

When you recognize and return to your essence, you can see with your heart, you can live in this world with a perception of love, which is your nature. Your life flourishes, your health is optimized, your relationships improve, and your finances take a

180-degree turn. All this happens because you are living in your essence, in what makes everything around you flourish. You already have everything you need to heal your life and your body. "You already have everything you need to be happy. Your real job is to do whatever it takes to realize this." -Geneen Roth.

The Brain in Your Heart

Living in current times is fascinating, as science and spirituality are increasingly coming together. Science is discovering more about the power of human beings to create a new reality for their health and in other areas of life. In 1999, NASA built a satellite and sent it into space to measure energy fields that we cannot see with our eyes. It is called the Chandra Observatory[8] and in 2019, they celebrated twenty years of its launch. This satellite provides invaluable information that explains that space is not empty, as we previously thought. There is an energy structure that connects everything.

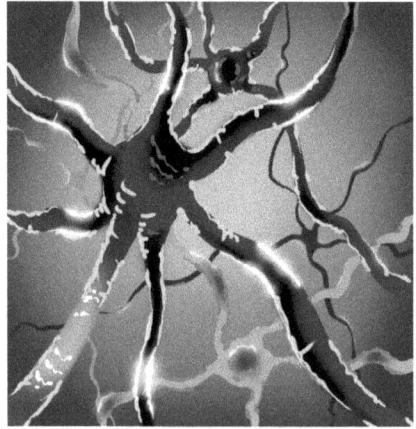

By looking at the images, you can appreciate that the space in the universe is like a connected network. What is significant is that this structure, and how energy aligns and connects in space, is similar to the way neurons in the brain align and connect. Science identified that the energy in our biology is connected with the energy of the universe[9]. Since everything you think, feel and create is energy, it has an innate connection to and effect on the universe. Science states that all possibilities already exist in the field of quantum energy[10].

Since our bodies are made of quantum particles[11], all the possibilities are already available to you, you just have to connect with that frequency. When you visualize your dreams with your mind and sincerely believe them in your heart, you bring those opportunities to life. The heart is vital, as it also has nerve cells; this is described as "the brain in your heart." Your mind creates the image of what you long for, but it is your heart that makes it come true in your life.

Patients who experience instant remissions show something in common: they are people who visualize their body as already healed and believe in their innate or divine power. As human beings, we complicate things by always seeking logic and thinking linearly without accepting there is power in the energy that is not seen, that of the divine. That is why we struggle to believe it is possible to heal with it.

The same energy that is in space is in each of your cells. The power that sustains this universe is in you. **I know it might be difficult to understand, but the universe is in you.** That energy and power are love, which connects and sustains everything.

Your creative source is love, and it is in each of your cells. You are in a world of love, and you live surrounded by it.

The meaning of love is bigger than we can humanly imagine. If you just acknowledge this, your life will change. In my clinical experience, I see this truth very often. Patients who believe in the innate power of their bodies to heal with a heightened and full consciousness experience healing faster, some instantaneously. They connect and return to their essence.

Going through life without recognizing who you are is contrary to your nature and ultimately brings you pain. Valentín, a well-loved seventy-year-old patient, healed his neck's stage-four degeneration. Stage-four degeneration means that the spine has had chronic degenerative damage for over fifty years, there is severe nerve interference, the normal curvature is lost, and the intervertebral discs have collapsed.

Conventional medicine does not give much hope of regeneration to a patient presenting such an advanced condition. However, Valentín healed his neck 100% in a year and a half. At his age, Valentin has the neck of a fifteen-year-old.

Valentín's story was very different when he first visited me. What he wanted was any relief from his neck pain. He believed that what he needed was something external. After evaluating him and explaining his case, Valentín recognized that the condition of his spine and his nervous system was very deteriorated. He understood that what he needed was not just pain relief, but healing. The pain was not the issue; it was a signal that his body gave him to get to the root of the problem.

He followed all the recommendations I gave him, came to his adjustments as often as recommended, followed a healthy eating guide, and began exercising his body. However, the most important thing was that he learned that the power to heal was already in him, so he returned to his essence and believed in the innate power to heal.

Every morning, he visualized his healthy spine. He learned the language of his heart, of his essence, and felt compassion and love for his body. He could recognize and connect with his innate power to heal. At six months, we re-evaluated Valentín and found that his spine had healed 50%.

His other health conditions improved, his blood pressure was now normal, and he could stop taking all of his medications. After a year, we re-evaluated him and verified that his spine had now healed 100%. Now, he continues to enjoy his family, his travels and his favorite hobbies. Valentín went from fear of illness and pain to love and appreciation for life and his body. He stopped having thoughts and beliefs based on the fear of having to live with sickness his entire life and being limited by a diagnosis, his history, his past and his beliefs. He generated healing, because he recognized that life actually works for him and not against him. He went from having stage-four vertebral degeneration to having a totally healed neck.

I can share story after story of healing, just like Valentín's. Each story is different, but what all these patients have in common is that they return to their essence to trust the healing power that lies within them. They are patients who follow recommendations to the letter because they believe, without a doubt, that their healing is possible.

Many people have to go through seriously difficult situations before raising their consciousness and returning to their essence; however, any circumstance that makes you wake up and connect with your essence is a blessing.

You were created to be healthy and complete in every area of your life. You were born to reflect your essence of love and our creator's power. By awakening to this new awareness and returning to your essence, your nature, you will allow others to do the same. By getting rid of fear, your very presence will free others. This is wonderful, right?

So, how can you put the power of love into practice within yourself? How do you find the power of your essence? Think about your current life or reality. Most likely, you have a tendency to divide your life into parts. You divide your personal and family life from your work or professional life. However, your essence is an important part of you, and it must be present equally in all facets of your life.

Do not judge the thoughts that threaten to overwhelm you as you examine the current state of your reality. Maybe there are areas in your life that you don't like. Just take a minute to observe yourself in every facet of your life. See yourself as a source of love and light as a parent, child, professional in your work, leader of your community. Visualize your essence of love in each of the areas of your life. Flood each of your relationships with your essence.

See the innocence in the people you interact with day to day and see yourself in them. Most likely, they do not think like you. Accept them for who they are, and not for what they do or think. This will replenish your sense of peace and heal all kinds of relationships. Each person is doing what they think is right at that moment, according to their level of consciousness.

In this same vein, see your body with love. If there is an area on your body that needs to heal, put your hand there and put the other on your heart. **Visualize love healing your body.** Feel love and compassion for your body. You are harmonizing your mind with your heart. It sounds amazing, and it feels amazing!

Miracles result from love. They occur naturally when you live in your essence, in your love. The true miracle is noticing how you returned to your essence.

"If we want to know what we were born for, we must first know how we were born: as the virtuous caretakers of the planet

designed fundamentally to live as if living and loving are one."
- anonymous.

The Power to Create Is in Your Essence

Are you aware of your power's magnitude? How do you use this power? Are you creating consciously? We all create our reality, even if we are not aware. You have the power to create your life and health.

Rumi, one of the most widely read poets, wrote: "You suppose you are the problem. But you are the cure. You suppose you are the lock on the door. But you are the key that opens it."

Please read this carefully. You return to your essence of love by raising your consciousness and living in the present, where you align yourself with your creative power. It is like when you want to tune in to your favorite radio station; you have to find the right frequency to hear it. You can not hear it if you are at another station.

You have the power of God and the universe to create a better reality. Live fully concious in the present. This is the key.

To communicate this concept more clearly, I share with you a beautiful and powerful experience. My chiropractic practice changed radically the moment I raised my consciousness, when I gave my full attention only to the patient in front of me and my focus was totally on their healing, visualizing the perfection of their body, and recognizing that my essence is love. I visualized my heart and hands radiating love to that patient, literally. Then everything changed. I saw changes in patients in more meaningful ways.

I always remember Connor, a little boy only seven years old. His mother brought him to our office for his eczema condition. For this mom, our office was her last resort, and she could not imagine how a chiropractor could help her son with skin problems. It was very moving to look at his little arms and the back of his knees, looking so red from the inflammation that affected his skin.

That day, I carefully evaluated Connor and next I explained the results to his mother. Then, we began his chiropractic care. Before adjusting his spine, I visualized his body, especially his skin, in complete health. As I put my hands on his spine, I could see with my heart the innate power of his body to heal. My heart exuded compassion for this child who came seeking help.

I adjusted the areas of his spine with a high level of neurological interference, and my priority at the moment was to be present and let the innate, healing power of his body flow. When I finished, I looked him in the eye and explained what he had to do at home. The instructions for Connor were simple:

"When you are in your room, alone and calm, you will speak with your body. You will tell your little arms and knees that you love them. You are going to send them love and you are going to give them permission to heal. Do this whenever you can, Connor."

Two days later, his mother returned with an amazed look on her face. This time she brought not only Connor, but three more children as well. Connor and his brothers got very moving results. I am excited to see how open children are to believe, as it is easier for them to see beyond what's external.

Just as Connor did, patients woke up and realized that health comes from the inside out, not from medicine or something external. I connected with patients in a deeper way. I understood I was connecting with their very essence. My focus was not on the physical limitations the patient presented, but on the innate power that heals their body. I adjusted their spines not only with my hands but also with my heart and a higher consciousness.

What I once could have only imagined today is a beautiful reality in my life. I live each day in love with the innate power of each patient to create their new reality, both in their health and in other areas of their life.

After evaluating the results of the well-known *Human Genome* project, leading scientists such as David Baltimore, one of the most recognized geneticists and a winner of the Nobel Prize, claim that your biology's complexity and the power of your consciousness cannot be attributed to your genetics[12].

It is important that you return to your essence. There lies the healing power that goes above your genes, age, or gender.

How do you apply this creative power in your daily life? Is there any part of your body that needs to heal? Maybe it is your liver, stomach, spine, heart, skin, intestines, or something else. When you wake up in the morning, even without getting out of bed, visualize that part of your body in a healed state. Recognize that there are millions of new cells in your body every day waiting for your brain's command to know what they are going to create. Imagine that army of new cells wondering, what are we going to create today?

Do not think that it is just another day of living with the same condition. It does not have to be that way. If your first thoughts in the morning are: "again with this arthritis pain in my hands," you are telling the thousands of new cells to keep forming more of the same, more arthritis in your hands, more pain. It is very important that you understand that your words and thoughts are energy that your body listens to. Your body continually renews itself and seeks this power in you. You can create a new reality in your health or in any other area of your life at any point in time. The power to create is in your essence.

I'll briefly describe an exercise that can help you. Read it and then put it into practice.

When you wake up in the morning, even in your bed, take a few minutes to flood your body with your essence of love. Close your eyes and breathe deeply. Just watch your breath. You do not have to be a meditation expert or a monk to have tremendous results. **Meditating is simply being present.** Have a feeling of compassion and love for your body, and visualize it as healthy. Put your mind to the desired result as if it already happened. Your body follows the instructions of your intention. Continue that practice every day. Each of the cells in your body will vibrate very differently.

Your subconscious is much faster than your conscious mind and is programmed with the beliefs you've had since childhood. By making this exercise a habit in your life, you will change your subconscious. Do not worry about understanding the complexity of all the different reactions that you are creating within your body while doing this practice. Just trust in the great power it possesses and how it allows you to heal yourself. Visualize your body in its healthy state, trust in the innate power to heal and love your body intensely. Do it. You will see where this practice will take you. Your mornings will have a new meaning.

Just as you bathe, comb your hair, and select what to wear before leaving your house, it is important that you also take time in the morning to connect your mind with your body and spirit before starting your daily tasks. You will see that everything you do early in the morning, before leaving your house, can change your day, your health, and your life.

There is a connection between your state of consciousness, your perception, and what you experience as your reality. Your mind has been limited to interpreting different events in certain ways according to what you experienced in the past. Your perception creates your reality. How your mind deciphers something establishes how you respond or react to things or events that happen around you.

I remember experiencing one of the most catastrophic events in the history of Puerto Rico, the famous Hurricane Maria which passed right through this beloved island. The first days after the hurricane, it seemed as if a bomb had just exploded. Almost everything that was green before had died. Imagine, a Caribbean island without vegetation.

It was moving and shocking to see these changes in nature, but the most moving thing was to see how each person's life changed according to what they were perceiving. Many perceived the hurricane only as a tragedy, while others saw it as an opportunity to make changes, to reinvent themselves. Their thoughts were more elevated than their current situation.

I have never experienced a catastrophic event of this magnitude before. I learned so much from the palm trees! It was impressive to see them for hours and hours, bending completely to the ground with each gust of wind, but then they would rise again, as if they had an internal spring helping them. Their ability to bend and be one with the changes of the storm allowed them to survive. In the same way, resilience in the face of adversity helps you cope with sudden changes and be able to be calm again.

The way you experience your reality is not defined by the events that happen to you, but by the way you perceive and react to those events. Possibly, you have had moments in which you think you live captive in your own reality, without being aware of your contribution to that current situation.

You may believe that because you are sixty years old, you can no longer do the things you used to enjoy doing, like practicing your favorite sport, or traveling the world, or maybe learning something new like playing an instrument or learning a new dance. Perhaps you tell yourself that your aches and pains are a product of your age and you consider that it's normal to live sick and taking medications for the rest of your life. Maybe you're young, but you are already having beliefs that limit your expression of life.

What are your limiting beliefs? Realize that by holding onto these beliefs, you allow your mind to trap you.

I hope you can create consciously, choosing your thoughts and letting go of the beliefs that you have held and have ruled your mind and life for so many years.

Your Mind's Energy

Remember that your thoughts are energy. They are linked to the invisible part of reality, the part that controls the creation of the physical world, the world that you experience with your five senses. When you think and feel, you are transmitting energy.

You do not see it physically, just as you cannot see the energy that turns on the light in your house.

Science increasingly studies the relationship of energy with matter. Everything is energy, what we can and cannot see with our eyes. If you look inside an atom, you could see that what is there is energy. The atom is not how you remember it in your physics books. If you look for it again, you see it is described as waves of energy[13].

Have you ever noticed how the atmosphere of a place changes when you enter? For example, have you ever entered a business when it's quite empty, but after your arrival everything changes and little by little people arrive until suddenly it is completely full? This is not by chance, everything responds to the energy you brought to that place.

Your thoughts and feelings' energy create your body and the external world, and I mean the material, tangible world you can see with your eyes. By returning to your essence of love, you can change your thoughts and feelings, and thus transform how your life manifests. This is something radically new for many, and perhaps for you too. Not understanding your essence makes you feel separated from society, purposeless and powerless.

The world that you can physically see was formed by what you cannot see with your eyes. For example, think about what had to happen at the time of your conception. What force was present for you to be conceived? Could someone see that creative power? That creative power is in you. It is you. It is your essence. You are not separate from this creative power, but you cannot see that power that gives life and shape to tangible things with your physical eyes.

The power to create is in your essence. You were born with the right to create your life and your health.

You are here now, in this time and place. Your presence makes a difference on this Earth. Perhaps you live separated from this creative force by not understanding your essence. Your Creator made you in its image. Its qualities are yours, that is your magnificence. **Being aware of who you are is the key to a long life.** Joy, laughter, benevolence and compassion will extend your life, because those are the qualities of your Creator. Return to your essence, reconnect with this creative power.

To Be and to Do – The Mary and Martha in You

Do you remember or have you heard the Bible story where Jesus visits Martha and Mary's house? I remember listening to this story as a child and imagining Jesus sitting and talking with Mary. Enjoying Jesus' visit, she gave him her full attention as they sat together. Nothing was more important than paying attention to the teacher visiting her home. Wow, imagine that! Without a doubt, Mary enjoyed that moment with all her heart.

Martha, on the other hand, was very anxious and preoccupied with all of her household chores. I imagine her cooking in a hurry and, when she saw her sister Mary sitting, attentive to Jesus, she got upset because she was not helping her. Imagine Martha angrily asking Jesus, "Why do you not tell my sister to help me?". Jesus answered Martha in a way that she did not expect. "Martha, Martha," the Lord answered, "you are worried and upset about many things, but few things are needed—or indeed only one. Mary has chosen what is better, and it will not be taken away from her." Luke 10: 41-42.

Can you relate to Martha when you think that you always have something to do? Or maybe you're always talking about something you have to do, or that you need someone to do, instead of just being present with those around you, your partner, children, or parents. Have you ever taken the time to enjoy love, which is the essence that you share with them?

Mary and Martha's phases are *being* and *doing*.

Being is primary. *Doing* is secondary. **We are primarily living beings, not living "doings".** This continues to be one of the biggest lessons in my life.

These two aspects are always in your life - *being* and *doing*. Many people only know the *doing* and are completely unaware of their *being*. Many people learn to identify entirely with *doing*, and this includes thinking. Maybe you have not seen it like that, but when you think, you are doing something.

Now you can see how many live in a state of constant anxiety, worry, and stress, totally ignoring the possibility of just *being*. When you analyze Jesus and his life, you realize that his main teaching was to teach us to *be*.

If you, like many people, identify with your thoughts, you become captured by them. You get caught up in thinking and *doing*. You constantly think about what comes next, what else you have to do, different bills to pay, your next doctor's appointment, your son's field trip, your daughter's special assignment, your next project, and so on.

Each time, you disconnect more from the deepest dimension in you, from the essence of who you are. You are not even aware of its existence. You stay looking at the world from a perspective that is outside of your body, of your essence, of your first home.

Even before you go to sleep, you keep asking yourself, what else do I have to do? What else do I have to think about? What is the first thing I have to do in the morning? And if that were not enough, you look at the evening news or social media to keep thinking. **No wonder so many people struggle to sleep! It's because they are constantly thinking and doing and, thus, can not be free.**

I can already hear you ask, "So then, I should do nothing?" That is not it. Your essence is in the state of *being*. It is where you recharge your battery in order to *do*. Jesus meant that the priority was to *be*, and everything else is secondary. You can see Martha and Mary as one human being. We all have a part of Martha and Mary in us, and we can be both.

Find the balance between *being* and *doing* to have health, happiness, and fulfilment in every area of your life.

If you only live in the state of *doing*, then you identify with what you do and think, and in the same way, you identify with the ego. The ego is who you think you are. It is the "fake" you. The ego is to recognize yourself by what your mind tells you according to the image you have of yourself, your thoughts, the things you do, your achievements or what you want to achieve or with your occupation. You are not your mind or what you think, or the profession or occupation that you exercise. Realize that the real you is much more than any material thing or external achievement.

Being, as a priority, is not a concept that I expect you to understand fully just by reading this book; it is something that requires experience to be understood. *Being* is what you learn when you are alert, living in the moment, when you are present in stillness.

The next time you are in bed, just before sleeping, pay attention to your breathing. Can you feel your lungs? Do not analyze or think: be fully aware, be one with your body, recognize how it feels to be alive. Can you feel your right hand without touching it? Do you know where it is? Can you feel its pulsations? I love how in Psalms 46:10, the Bible tells us that in stillness we know God, our Creator, or your creative source, whatever you want to call it. God is much more than a concept or a word.

To recognize *being* as a priority is the most important thing in your life, your state of consciousness. Discover that internal space within yourself where you are aware and alert, but not thinking. Immense power lies in that internal space. When you start this practice, it may seem strange to you and perhaps you will feel that nothing is happening and it makes little sense. But, when you go to the most intimate depths of yourself, you realize you are in your state of *being*. Your presence will recognize your identity of consciousness and you will return to your essence.

I vividly remember when, from a young age, I discovered the enormous power of the dimension of *being* in stillness. I believe that the pain of leaving my home and my country at an early age led me to this great lesson. Perhaps I did not understand this dimension of *being* in its totality, but it awakened in me a feeling of life, of unequaled joy. It led me to understand that this is where true power lies, where you are one with your Creator. It is living in heaven on Earth.

One of my favorite authors, Eckhart Tolle, wrote two powerful books: *The Power of Now* and *A New Earth*. I recommend them. They will help you understand the power of being and living consciously in the present moment.

The Balance Between *Being* and *Doing*

The objective is that you achieve *being* and *doing* at the same time in your daily life: at work, school, home, and in your moments of recreation. When you do or think, do not let your presence of *being* be pushed to the side. Then you will not get completely lost in your thoughts or actions.

A simple and everyday example would be when you go for a walk. Wherever you go, make sure you're present in that daily process. Feel your legs move, listen to your breath, feel the air, see the surrounding abundance. Enjoy every step. Do not get lost just thinking about where you are going.

Do this with every daily task, no matter how mundane it may seem. Live life being consciously present. Life will become full of enjoyment if you just awaken to your essence of *being*. Have you ever noticed how you feel when you look into the eyes of a child or a pet? They are more present in the dimension of *being*, and that is why they transmit peace to you.

Another example that means a lot to me has to do with parenting. If you have young children, you know that going through the whole routine to take your children to school can be exhausting. Get up in the early morning, make breakfast, finish packing their lunch boxes, put their backpacks in the car, wake up your kids and get them ready for their school day, and then drive through heavy traffic to school. Already at eight in the morning, you feel as if you have run a marathon. While doing all those everyday tasks, are you conscious? Are you present? Is your essence of *being* present in your daily tasks?

Do not get lost just in *doing*. Enjoy being able to dress your children, to brush and style their hair. The road to school can be a time of connection with your children that they will never forget and, if they fall asleep, enjoy watching the sunrise.

Do not lose that feeling of witnessing the miracles in everyday life. Do not get lost in the doing.

It is important to recognize the almost secret identity of the ego. It is known for being a continuous feeling of lacking, insufficiency, and always wanting more. Your mind creates the ego and always seeks to protect and enhance its identity. The ego feels challenged if it loses something or if it does not get what it wanted for the future. It also feels challenged when you perceive that other people have more or better material things. It's intimidated by perceiving others as more powerful, smarter, or better looking.

If you get your identity through what your ego identifies with, you will compare yourself to others frequently. Some days you'll feel that you are better than others, other days you feel you are worse. It all depends on what happens outside of yourself and what other people think, do, or have.

The ego always wants more. It is never satisfied. It never frees you from that state of dissatisfaction. You can externalize your desires and have the things you want to have and be, in which there is no harm. **It is your privilege to create the life you long for.** But, if you do not return to your essence, you can spend your life looking for yourself in other things or people.

You will continually seek fulfillment, but you can never experience it; frustration will come even if you get what you want, because there will always be something more to wish for if you are not in connection with your essence and your state of *being*. It works the other way around: first you must return to your essence and then the rest (material things) will come to you. Things or people in the future do not give fulfillment to you. Fulfillment results from living in the present, being aware of your true essence.

Your Connection With Your Essence Dissipates the Ego

Depriving yourself of the dimension of *being* will deprive you of what is most essential. It is poignant to see that many still do not know their own essence. What do I mean? When you look at the behavior of people around you, or in other parts of the world, you can see that their lives are rooted in things that happen to others and what they hear about in the news. Anxiety and anguish overshadow their lives, and they are constantly reacting to circumstances.

Surely you know of people who, when they lose material things that identified them, such as their fame, money, and reputation, lose themselves completely and deprive themselves of living because it was all they knew. They associated their identity and sense of *being* only with the material world. By losing what was material, they totally lose themselves or, on the contrary, they awaken to a higher consciousness and find their essence or their dimension of *being*.

There is a hidden wealth in any illness, misfortune or disaster. They have the potential to teach you to look inward; they push you to discover a higher consciousness that invites you to transcend. There is no better example than the global crisis we are experiencing with COVID-19; it invites us to change and transcend.

If nothing is random, what is the reason for the current situation? What changes is this pandemic asking of us? You can recognize that it calls us to look within, to return to our essence and thus raise our consciousness. Diseases come to us when we do not inhabit our first home, our essence. We will see that the fruitful behavior and actions of humanity will result from a heightened consciousness. "When you come out of the storm, you won't be the same person who walked in. That's what this storm's all about." - Haruki Murakami.

Human beings identify with all material things. There is nothing wrong with having and appreciating the things that we have, enjoy, and surround us. What does not help us is to identify ourselves or establish our value based on them; Nothing that comes into our lives is permanent.

Recently, I heard the story of a young mother who, despite the danger posed by continuing to live at home because of the effects of many earthquakes in the region where she lives, refused to leave. Her house was not safe. Several people encouraged her to evacuate for her safety and that of her son, but the mother insisted on staying. When asked why she refused to vacate, she replied she did not want to leave her new television set. She clung strongly to this material possession because she identified with it, to such a level that her safety and that of her son became secondary.

The most important thing to recognize in your life is the transcendental aspect of *being* at all times. To begin, find where you can stop thinking and where you can enjoy those little lapses of pure presence. Recognize those moments when you are just observing something, without thinking; there you will feel your *being*.

If you take the time to observe, you will see that life comprises a succession of small events. The big events that you expect for days, months, or years do not shape most of your life. Joy and fulfillment come from being aware of the little things. You can look at the sky without having to analyze it, just observe it and absorb all its abundance.

Catch yourself just observing more often, have moments like those more frequently during the day. You will return to your essence and soon your essence will shine throughout your physique and in everything you do.

You will have a tangible body as long as you are on this planet. Your body identifies itself with matter, with all that is physical. But, as you practice being consciously present and experiencing your dimension of *being*, your essential identity will radiate your physical identity with its light.

I recently saw a cute movie, *Star girl*, and it describes this. It is the story of a teenage girl who lives an extraordinary life, because she is connected with her dimension of *being*. The surrounding people can see her essence's light.

The power to heal your mental,spiritual, and physical health lies in your return to your essence. You will realize that it is already in you. It is not a power that seeks to control, but liberates - it is the power of life itself.

Meditation - A Magnificent Tool

"The intuitive mind is a sacred gift and the rational mind a faithful servant. We have created a society that honors the servant by completely forgetting about the gift." -Bob Samples, *The*

Metaphoric Mind: A Celebration of Creative Consciousness. The power of intuition is a gift like no other. I firmly believe that, as a society, we are waking up to this truth. Meditation strengthens intuition.

Many may think that it is difficult to meditate; initially, your mind does not like it. When you consciously quiet your body, your mind knows that it will also have to quiet down, that it cannot continue to be the controlling boss, it cannot rule. If your mind directs you, your life gets filled with suffering, as it can be a terrible boss. When you meditate, your mind is not the boss, your *being* is in charge. You are no longer a slave to your mind. **By becoming a more meditative person, your mind will become a wonderful instrument.**

Meditation is not about doing something specific. The essence of meditating is merely not trying to get anywhere. It is to be where you already are, to experience your *being* in the here and now.

True meditation is the realization of your *being*. It is not about meditating. It is just *being*. There lies the power.

You realize that the most liberating thing gives you satisfaction. It is like a fragrance that you really enjoy on yourself. You can get to where it becomes one of your habits and you meditate endlessly. You will *do* and *be* in balance. It means that in everything you do, your essence of *being* is not lost: you drive your car and you are in your essence of *being*. You talk with a friend while you are in your essence of *being*. You recognize that, physically, you are there, living your everyday life, and at the same time, you express your dimension of *being* in your daily life.

The power to heal your life and your health is already in you, but it hides behind your noisy mind and the noisy world that incessantly insists and harasses you with physical things that require your attention. Your mind overwhelms you, because every moment it asks you for more attention. And so, you continue to identify your reality with your overwhelmed mind, to perceive everything that happens around you based on the condition of your thoughts.

This bombardment is even more intense today. Technology, social media, and other distractions bog your mind down. There is a lot of unimportant information, mostly destructive and very negative. It is very easy to abandon the connection with your being.

Still, there is a change, a spiritual evolution; Many people are waking up and identifying less and less with the mind and ego, with material goods, and consumerism.

Without a doubt, you can have the material things that you want and long for in any area, but if you do not connect with your essence of being, fulfillment and satisfaction will not come. "But seek first his kingdom and his righteousness, and all these things will be given to you as well." (Matthew 6:33). You might think that the kingdom of God is far from you, separate. You look up at the sky and think it is up there. What the word "kingdom" refers to is the inner space you connect to when you are still, when you seek that transcendental part or space. Luke 17:21 says, "[...] because the kingdom of God is in your midst." The kingdom is in you, because it refers to that transcendental space.

Stillness

It is in stillness that you can see your Creator and recognize that you are an extension of his power and love. Being made in the image of your Creator means you reflect your Creator. It is there that you realize your Creator is not a linear concept. Similarly, your body can heal and regenerate itself in stillness.

Practice this: watch how you breathe, notice the air going into your lungs and the air coming out of them, feel it, appreciate the intervals between each breath. This is an excellent relaxation technique. Understand that this exercise, as simple as it may seem, invites your entire body to heal and perform each of its functions optimally. You are signaling your brain that all is well, and thus your cells will fill with a sense of life.

This is a simple way to meditate. Contemplate your breath. Sometimes thoughts will come, but just return your attention to your breath. There are few things as valuable and, at the same time, so undervalued as your breath. Cultivate this practice in your daily life.

When you have a few minutes, calm your mind. It will increase your effectiveness when you need to think. It will contribute to your mental clarity; your thoughts will be more efficient, elevated, powerful, intelligent, concrete and defined. You will connect with the most intimate depths of yourself, with unconditional awareness and the power that keeps you alive and breathing. Your mind will not be wandering without focus. It is like what happens when you turn off your computer after long hours of use and having dozens of windows open at the same time; you notice that restarting your computer makes you perform better. This practice is truly significant.

Having the ability to rise above thought without leaving your consciousness is a precious thing. It is a spiritual awakening that is not about religion, but about recognizing the dimension of *being* and consciousness in you, which was always there, but you had overlooked it.

Think of a time when you felt fully alive. I am sure you have experienced it. It is a moment where you felt an abundant amount of joy and peace. Realize that, in those moments, you thought little. They are moments where you were, in your essence, more connected to your dimension of *being*.

Thinking is a very useful and indispensable property, as long as your thoughts do not dominate you. The mind is a great tool for creating. But if it is your mind that uses you, you become its prisoner. Your mind dominates you if you totally identify with your thoughts.

People may feel like they cease to exist when they let go of their thoughts, because they are addicted to thinking.

I believe that one of the biggest addictions is not the addiction to medicines, drugs, alcohol, cigarettes, or food: it is the addiction to thinking. When you cannot stop, thoughts pretend to be more powerful than you and dominate you.

You can create problems in your mind and consequently bring them to reality. You can create obstacles where there are none, in your health and in other areas of your life. Analyze how much stress you generate through your excessive, unnecessary thoughts, without clear intention or focus. Many people cause unhappiness in their lives by their unconscious mental activity, loaded with judgments and inadequate interpretations of other people and their circumstances.

When you are still, you recognize two aspects within you: *being* and *doing*, or Mary and Martha. You are a person and also an expression of a consciousness that goes beyond yourself. If you are not looking for an internal and intimate space of stillness, of not thinking, nothing can satisfy you. You will have temporary satisfactions, but not permanent ones. There is no external thing that can satisfy you completely. There are no achievements, riches, people, or physical health that give you permanent satisfaction. The inner space in stillness frees you and heals you.

CONSTRUCT #3:

A Healed Mind – an Admirable Gift

The Quality of Your Mind

I told you that your mind has to be healthy and not dominate your life in order to be a tool for creating your new reality. You cannot have a troubled mind to achieve your goal. It is like wanting to cook up a delicious recipe. You know you can do it, but the ingredients you have are not of good quality and you do not have the oven you need, or the kitchen tools to achieve your recipe.

What is the quality of your mind? Are you aware of the state of your mind? This is the first step. My intention in this chapter is to help you understand how mental patterns are constantly creating your life experiences-the good ones and the not so good ones. I want to help you understand how mental patterns contribute to your health or illness.

I love Louise L. Hay's definition of health: "Good health is having no fatigue; having a good appetite; going to sleep and awakening easily; having a good memory; having good humor; having precision in thought and action; and being honest, humble, grateful, and loving. How healthy are you?"[14]

I hope you understand that true healing is not only physical, but begins by returning to yourself and connecting with your essence. When your consciousness' healing energy is flowing through your mind and heart, then you can heal physically.

Healing will occur when you give your body permission to heal.

Let me ask you, do you really want to heal? Are you willing to open your heart and mind to the recommendations you read in this book? The power to heal is already in you. My job is merely to be a facilitator, to help you recognize that the doctor is in you. Ram Dass wrote in his book, *Be Here Now,* *"You don't need to go anywhere else to find what you're seeking"* In other words, you do not have to go anywhere else to find what you are looking for. You have everything you are looking for. It has been there the whole time and, if you give it the opportunity, you will recognize it.

What Is Sickness?

In my opinion, disease is part of a lesson. It is vital that you do not just complain and say, "I want this disease to go away." That will not generate the healing you seek and you will not learn the lesson, either. I am not trying to condemn or create guilt; I just want you to bring to the surface what needs to be exposed. Disease may happen because you are completely disconnected or do not recognize what is happening in your mind and your body. **Many people only pay attention to their bodies when illness strikes.**

Healing does not mean returning to the state you were in previously. Healing means being more aware than before, being closer to your Creator. Have you ever listened to your body? I love one of the most heard and read phrases by Shakti Gawain in her book *The Four Levels of Healing*: "Our bodies communicate with us clearly and specifically, if we are only willing to listen to them."

This is your time to heal. It is the time to make your life and your body complete. Within you there is a center of wisdom. When you are ready to make positive changes in your life, you will attract everything you need to help you.

Internal Dialogue

Your physical body reflects your internal dialogue. It is a mirror of your thoughts and beliefs. Each of your cells responds to every thought and word. Imagine your cells as little people who work together to carry out their different functions, and what determines their future is the internal environment where they live, which is created by your dialogue. What is your internal dialogue? Think for a moment. What do you constantly tell yourself? What do you say to your body on a day-to-day basis?

Analyze for a moment your internal dialogue from yesterday and determine if that internal dialogue had something to do with your reality today. I will give you a common example that perhaps has happened to you. You wake up in the morning already overwhelmed, rushing to get out of the house before the traffic picks up. You are in a rush to get to work on time. Before getting into your car, you notice that the left tire is flat. Everything in your mind becomes clouded, your heart beats louder, and you think and believe that your day has been completely ruined. You tell yourself that these things always happen to you, that you have the worst luck, and thus you create your reality according to how you perceive your car's empty tire. Your mind stayed on the flat tire all day. Your spirits lowered. That event dictated the rest of your day. Ram Dass wrote in *Experiments in Truth*, "Taking something too seriously does not make it go away. In fact, it makes the situation a little worse."

Now, on the contrary, imagine just accepting what happened. You have a flat tire, you cannot change that fact. It is common for tires to go flat from time to time. Just by accepting the little things that happen, you create your inner peace and, peacefully, you can find answers to those little situations. You do not make up a mental story; you accept what happened and move on.

You think clearly. You know that your day is not determined by that event, and you can imagine that somehow God, your Creator, or the universe is protecting you from something. Something bigger than your situation guides you. Everything happens for a reason. You ask for an Uber or call a friend and you get to your work calmly. Maybe you were supposed to meet the Uber driver, or see the friend who can help you. You did not create an unreal story in your mind. Let every day teach you a new lesson. Allow life to flow through you and for each day to be your teacher.

Studies estimate that we have around 60,000 to 70,000 thoughts a day, of which 90% are the same as yesterday, and the previous week, and the previous year. Maybe you have asked yourself, why does my life stay the same? The answer is clear: if your thoughts remain the same, your emotions and actions will remain the same. I ask you again, what has been your internal dialogue? Write it here:

Internal dialogue about health:

Internal dialogue about relationships:

Internal dialogue about personal finance:

You can look at people's faces and see that they show the internal dialogue they carry throughout their lives. I reiterate that **your privilege and right on this Earth is to have complete health and to be fulfilled in every area of your life.**

By studying the origin of most diseases, we recognize we create them ourselves[15]. I do not mean that you consciously wanted it. You did not say, "I want to have diabetes" or "I want to have this heart condition." But, you created a mental environment where disease occurs and grows.

Your cells are like people who respond to the environment they are in, which is determined by what you think and say. If your internal dialogue is negative and nonconstructive, you should know that your internal environment is a place where disease can naturally occur and grow. You are responsible for every experience in your life. By changing the perception of your subconscious, you will change your reality.

You create each experience with your thoughts and your words. Start being an observer of your thoughts. Learn to look at them in a detached manner. This will be a new beginning that will revolutionize your life and your health.

Ask yourself: is this thought that I am having one that builds or destroys me? Is it a thought that heals me or does it make me sick? Do I want this thought to shape my future?

Maybe you wake up in the morning thinking that everything is the same, that your health is not improving, or that you can never buy your own house with the current economy. Or, perhaps you think you cannot start that business you have always wanted, that you are not ready yet. Henry Ford used to say, "Whether you think you can or you think you can't, you're right.

Maybe you think you do not choose your thoughts, that they just come to you, but they do not. You have become used to not seeing them consciously, but you have the power to choose what you think. Start choosing thoughts that help create an environment where your body can heal. Remember that your internal dialogue is creating your reality, today and tomorrow, because your internal dialogue becomes the environment of your cells.

Your internal dialogue dictates your energetic vibration, and the universe responds to it.

Your Parents and Your Thinking Model

"It is very difficult to grow, because it is difficult to let go of the models of ourselves in which we invest so much." -Ram Dass, *One-Liners: A Mini-Manual for Spiritual Life.*

When you were little, you learned systems or ways of thinking and grew to see life according to them. You can look back and see that your experiences reflect what you believe to be true. Growing up, you might blame your parents for something they taught you or did not teach you. But in reality, nothing happens by chance and your parents are the ideal ones to teach you something specific that you need to learn for the future. Keep in mind that your parents were doing the best they could with what they were taught as children.

No matter how long you have had a disease or a problem, the source of power is in the present, today. What you choose to think, believe, and say now creates your future. You choose your thoughts. Maybe you believe this is not the case, because you have had the same thoughts for a long time. It is possible that you won't allow healthy and positive thoughts about yourself to surface. Likewise, you can refuse to accept harmful thoughts from yourself.

The Four Most Dangerous Thought Models for Your Life and Health

"Let's not forget that the little emotions are the great captains of our lives and we obey them without knowing it." - Vincent Van Gogh.

Thoughts are the origin of your emotions. When you think something, the dendrites within your brain exchange information through neuropeptides. This generates emotions you feel in your body, and those emotions create behaviors. So the way you behave is because of something very profound.

Famous psychiatrist Sigmund Freud compared the iceberg to the human mind. The tip of the iceberg, which is about 15% of the whole, is all you see. This represents your actions, behavior, and reality. The 85% that cannot be seen is the part that is submerged in water. This deep part represents your thoughts and your emotions. Most of the things you think and do are the product of habits that you do unconsciously, a product of the subconscious.

I want to bring up some thoughts that affect your life the most, because they create an internal environment where disease can occur and grow. **I describe below the four models of thinking that I consider the most harmful.** These thought patterns come from not being present or paying attention to your mind. You realize that these four thought patterns come from not living in the present, but in the past or future.

1) Fear

Remember, love is what we are born with, and fear is what we learn as we grow. Fear rules most of the population. Fear comes from not believing that you deserve to live fully.

Fear is the absence of love, just as darkness is the absence of light. Fear is unconsciously asking for and attracting into your life what you do not want to happen. Is there fear ingrained in your mind? Maybe it is fear of the future, of being alone or of being with people, fear of being judged, or of the opinion of others about you. There are those who are afraid of illness, failure, or success.

I know that most of us have experienced fear at some point in our lives, and it is common to feel it at certain times, but it is not normal and not healthy to live most of our lives with this feeling. Your cells grow, regenerate and can perform their functions optimally when you are under the perception of love, not in fear[16].

It is important that you identify what creates fear so that you can change your perception to one of love. What do I mean? A common example that most of us have experienced is feelings of fear before speaking to a group of people. I know from my experience; I have felt fear before speaking in public. However, I learned to look at fear, recognize it, and replace it with love. I hope you can do the same.

The next time you are afraid, look at your fear and acknowledge it. Just understand that it is there. Learn to look at fear from a higher level of understanding, and you will see how it will dissolve. Remember that the feeling is not you, and realize that you can change it.

It always amazes me to experience the contrast. In the middle of some public presentation, I fully enjoy myself, educating and empowering my patients, and I realize that, at my core, I am doing what I love.

Love will always have the power to free you from fear.

In his book *The Mind - Gut Connection*, Emeran Mayer, MD explains new discoveries about the connection between your mind and the digestive system. Constantly living under negative thoughts and feelings, such as fear, can create ulcers and colon problems. Realize that fear is a thought that can be changed. If you relax and recognize that life really works for you and not against you, it will be easier for you to heal. Living under the influence of fear is just surviving, always preparing for the worst to happen.

Think of your breathing, which is one of the most valuable thing humans have. You breathe without thinking, without being aware of your breathing, and you have had many breaths throughout your life. You assume that the oxygen for your next breath will be there. Likewise, you can believe and trust that the same power that makes you breathe cares for you throughout your physical life and that everything you need is already here for you. **Your longings and true desires are on the other side of fear.**

2) *The Shame and Guilt of the Past*

In 2001, a group of researchers led by Sally Dickerson from the University of California at Los Angeles (UCLA), demonstrated how shame increases the activity of cytokines in the blood. They took a group of students and studied how their opinions affect their immune system. They asked one part of the group to write about some experience they felt ashamed of, and the other part to write about some event that did not cause embarrassment.

The researchers found that the blood tests of the group that felt shame showed an increase in cytokine activity. Cytokines in the blood are a signal of inflammation in the body, indicating the presence of a disease. The more shame and guilt, the more cytokine activity in the blood. The more shame and guilt, the more inflammation in your body.

Shame and self-blame cause physical and chronic pain.

Many times, this feeling is so deep and ingrained that you do not realize it exists because it is in the subconscious. Shame or guilt for something from the past is a feeling that has no use, no benefits, and cannot change any situation. Only you can get out of the prison of shame or guilt. You can begin by saying and believing this affirmation: "I choose to accept myself as I am, I choose to love myself, and I forgive myself for being so hard on myself. I let go of all feelings of shame or guilt and I accept the fullness and happiness that life has in store for me."

3) Criticism

Like shame, criticism also creates patterns of inflammation in your blood.

Imagine your cells in their internal environment. Blood is the environment where they carry out their different functions. The quality of the environment in your blood determines the behavior of your cells, and is where they create health or disease. But, what initially determines the composition of your blood are your thought patterns.

The inflammation in your joints, hands, feet, shoulders, knees, etc., can come from being a perfectionist, from feeling the need to control every situation or every person. Self-criticism will bring more critical people into your life. Why do you want to be perfect? Why do you have such high standards? Why worry about trying to control everything and everyone? Let life flow through you.

There is a hidden power in accepting events, things, and people as they are.

You do not know what will happen later today, or tomorrow, or in a year. You cannot control every event. Trying to control events, things, or people creates a continuous environment of tension and stress within you.

There is enormous power in trusting and letting the power that gave you life take care of placing every event, thing, or person where they need to be. Trust, and see that you are cared for and guided. **Just for today, do not judge or criticize anything, any event or person, much less yourself. Do it for today.**

4) Resentment

Resentment is one of the most toxic feelings for your health and life. Physically, it weakens your immune system, giving pathogens a chance to reproduce and create diseases like cancer. Resentment wears out the body. Maybe you live carrying this feeling for something that happened a long time ago. **The past is over and you cannot change it, but you can change your thoughts and attitude about the past.**

The point where you have the most power is always in the present. It is crazy to punish yourself for something that happened in the past. You can be aware of this feeling and decide to change it. Do not let it invade your life and your body. Frederic Luskin, PHD, is a Stanford University researcher who studied the effects of forgiveness. He says that people who learn to forgive have better health.

Forgiveness is synonymous with canceling a debt and requires genuine love. The book *A Course in Miracles*, written by Helen

Schucman, teaches that all illnesses are because of a failure to forgive.

Forgiveness is liberating and healing.

It is vital that you are aware of and let go of those thought patterns that do not allow you to heal. Your perception of life and the Creator should support you, not hinder you. The universe fully supports your internal dialogue. Your subconscious mind recognizes everything you agree to believe as true. What you believe about yourself and about life becomes your truth. When you let go of harmful thought patterns, you will attract healing.

You can repeat this statement: "I am open and willing to change the pattern of thought that contributes to my illness, and I will trust and allow my body to heal." You may not fully understand how this is possible, but there is something in you that will recognize that you have what it takes to heal. You will understand that you contributed to this disease, but now you can bring back your power to heal.

You are much more than those negative thoughts and emotions in your mind, and you can observe them as separate entities from you. It is like a blaze of fire that goes out if you do not add fuel to it. Your negative thoughts and emotions go out if you don't keep feeding them.

You are not alone, nor lost, much less abandoned. Remember that you are one with the same power that created you, and this power gives you the opportunity to create your health and your life.

Mirror Exercise

This is an exercise I learned from Lisa Nichols that changed my life. It helped to reprogram my subconscious and to
create thought patterns according to the reality I want to
see in my life.

Every day, for thirty days, look in the mirror and say:

"(Your name), I love you and you are enough." (Five times.)

"(Your name), I admire these things about you: _____ ."
(Five things.)

"(Your name), I forgive you for: _____ ."
(Five things.)

"(Your name), I promise you: _____."
(Five things.)

_____

_____

_____

_____

_____

In this exercise, what you tell yourself every day may vary, and could be about events that happened in your life since childhood.

Your Changing Brain

I want to tell you a little about your brain, as the new scientific research surrounding the human brain is very inspiring and empowering. You may have heard the term "neuroplasticity." "Neuro" means brain. "Plasticity" means changeable.

Research on neuroplasticity started gaining traction in the 1960s. A great book on this topic is Norman Doidge's *The Brain that Changes Itself*, where he explores the most important research on neuroplasticity and shares amazing stories from people who have been able to use their minds to heal.

They proved that, at any age, your brain can change based on your new experiences. The previous belief was that the brain never changes, that what you were born with was all you had. They believed neurons do not reproduce after the first few years of life. New research shows that neurogenesis can continue throughout the human life.

To give you an idea, there are about 90 billion neurons in the human brain. The production of neurons, beginning in week three of human development, occurs at a rate of 250,000 per minute. Amazing, right?!

Visualize the neurons in a large row, one after another, with spaces in between, just as when you have to queue to pay for your purchase at the supermarket you leave a space between you and the person in front and another before the person behind. These spaces between your neurons are important, they are called synapses. When you were born you had approximately 2,500 synapses, at three years of age you had approximately 15,000 synapses, and by adulthood approximately 50% of these were removed because they were not used.

Your neurons form circuits or pathways, similar to highways and roads, that connect relatively distant areas of the brain or nervous system. Each circuit or path is associated with a particular action or behavior.

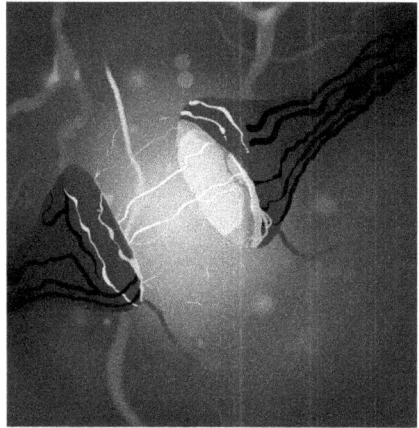

Now, visualize a well-marked circuit or path, which is known as a strong circuit. **Every time you think something you have thought before, or feel something you have felt before, you strengthen that circuit.** It is like going down the same road every day. These are your habits, circuits used continuously. They are strong circuits.

For example, in the morning you get up at the same time every day, on the same side of the bed, you go to the same bathroom, you bathe, you get dressed, you wash your mouth, you comb your hair, everything in that order because it is already a habit. You're on automatic, you don't even have to think about what you're doing. That is your subconscious in action.

Your subconscious contains your habits and represents 95% of what you do. Do you realize how important it is to become an observer of your thoughts and habits? Otherwise, you keep repeating the same thoughts and behaviors throughout your life without realizing it.

Your brain can change. Neuroplasticity gives us a new understanding of what it means to be human. We can reprogram, rearrange, and change our minds just by thinking. New thoughts and skills generate new circuits or paths. Repetition and practice strengthen these circuits until we create new habits, and thus the old circuits that are used less are weakened. It's like that old road that you no longer travel—eventually you forget that route. So, to have new circuits or paths, you need to practice your new way of thinking.

Literally, by continually choosing healthier and higher thoughts, you will create new circuits or pathways in your mind.

Therefore, it is vital that you reprogram your mind by choosing your thoughts early in the morning every day. **I emphasize the importance of becoming an observer of your thoughts. Remember, you have the power to choose them.** They don't come to you at random.

You may not see it because thinking in a certain way has become a habit. Observe and choose thoughts that go further than your current situation. All that holds you back or stops you are your thoughts, and it is up to you to change them. Everything in your life begins with your state of mind; abundance in your health, personal relationships and finances depends on your abundant thoughts.

Ask yourself: "This thought I have right now, does it heal me or make me sick? Does it build me or destroy me? Does it contribute to the new and better reality that I want to create?"

Here is an example in the area of health: when you wake up in the morning, think about what you want to see in your body. Remember that every day you have hundreds of millions of new cells ready to create health, and eliminate limiting thoughts that tie you to your past life. Change thoughts such as "this disease has no cure, I am just old, everything will remain the same, nothing will improve." Remember that your thoughts are creating your cell's internal environment. Tell your body what you expect of it, and trust it to do it.

Joe Dispenza is a renowned scientist who inspires with his healing testimony. In his book *The Placebo Is You*, he shows scientific evidence of how you can mold your brain and body with thoughts and emotions linked to your intention and the transcendental state that you experience.

Doctor and professor of neurology, Alvaro Pascual-Leone, M.D., a Harvard Medical School PhD, states that: "Mental training has the power to change our brain's physical structure."

He conducted a very interesting experiment with two groups of people. Group A practiced piano for two hours each day for five days; group B only imagined practicing piano, keeping their hands quiet for two hours a day for five days. The result was surprising—the two groups created the same changes in their brains.

You can activate new genes and create new circuits or pathways. Once you create a new circuit, your brain produces the necessary chemistry to form your feelings and emotions.

For example, imagine that you are reading a book on how to cook vegan food, and you are learning how healthy and effective it is for your body. Your brain stores this information in an area called the neocortex.

When you apply that information and start cooking at home, you strengthen those new circuits. You connect what you think with your actions, start eating healthy, and keep building a strong circuit in your brain. You have healthy feelings and emotions that foster well-being and love for your body, and teach your body what your mind understood with its intellect.

Another interesting study is Eleanor Maguire's, conducted in 1997. She observed changes in the taxi drivers' hippocampus associated with acquiring knowledge about the city of London. These taxi drivers showed a redistribution of gray matter. This research on the plasticity of the hippocampus interested scientists and the general public around the world. They found that the taxi driver's brain has a larger hippocampus and stores a detailed map of the city, while the brain of a musician has 130% more gray matter in the auditory cortex. This proves that the brain is like a muscle that grows with exercise.

How then can you create new and better circuits or paths, different from the ones you already have formed with thought patterns from your past that you know do not help you? **The answer is to be present, to give full attention to the present moment. This is the most important thing.**

Be consciously aware of your thoughts and decisions. Learn to observe your thoughts. I cannot emphasize how important this is. Start meditating. If you want, and if it helps you, you can remove the mystical aspect from meditation, or even rename it.

Instead of thinking that you have to belong to a group of yogis to meditate, have vast experience, or have the lights down low and a candle next to you, realize that you can meditate anywhere. It can happen in your vehicle before you start your day and rush out. Take two minutes before you hit the gas and just breathe. Be aware of your breathing, contemplate the place where you are, the tree or the building in front of you, look at the clouds, listen to the sounds of your car, just be present.

Remember, meditating is not doing something specific, but the opposite: it is being present and connecting with your being.

Meditation will bring you great changes. Meditation is going beyond your analytical mind, where you separate the external environment from your body, which is what controls your mind, and allowing your internal world to be more real than anything else.

To create change, learn to think bigger than your current life. My circumstances would never have allowed me to be a chiropractor, but I was able to think beyond my circumstances. I take this opportunity to tell you my story.

At fifteen, I left my native country in order to study, and at first I thought it would only be for a year. I still remember the letter I wrote to my dear parents before leaving. My home was full of love and security, and it gave me the strength to believe in what we cannot see. Even though I was young, my intuition told me I could study outside of my country. My conviction was very clear.

What at first I thought would be a year living in the state of Missouri turned into ten years of study. Within three or four years of living abroad, I discovered chiropractic. I knew I had to study this profession; I had no doubt that I would graduate as a doctor of chiropractic, although my circumstances indicated the opposite.

As a foreign student, I had no opportunities to get federal student loans. Chiropractic school was $7,000 to $10,000 per trimester, and I did twelve trimesters. Economically, it seemed not to be possible, but for reasons greater than what my analytical mind could see, I knew it would be. I could see myself as a chiropractor. So, I focused and started saving for the first trimester.

I remember my parents helped me some. The rest I saved from the part-time job I could have as a foreign student before entering chiropractic school. I got enough for the first trimester, but I had eleven more trimesters to go! It might seem illogical or perhaps unreasonable for me to jump into this, not knowing how I would do it for the next few trimesters, but I trusted my intuition and could see past my current situation.

In the middle of the first term, I had an idea: I wrote a letter where I explained my great desire to study, even though my financial situation did not seem to allow it. The intention of that letter was to obtain sponsorships from chiropractic doctors in the Missouri and Kansas City region, where there were many chiropractors, because the chiropractic school was in that region.

I sent hundreds and hundreds of letters. Do you know how many responses I got? None. I'm not denying it was daunting, but I was still confident. I could see that I would somehow continue into my second trimester, and I did. Fruits do not always come from the place where you sow, but from your intentions throughout the process. The fruit did not come directly from the letters I sent, but from the love and trust of a couple of people that wanted to help me grow.

An elderly couple from the church I was attending found out what I was doing and, without my asking, they helped me as co-signers to request a private student loan, which provided me with the financial resources to pay my second and third trimester. Before the end of the third trimester, one leader of that church offered to help me as a co-signer on another student loan so that I could continue. My heart swelled, and I accepted his help, which allowed me to complete another three terms.

Now I was already in the middle of my academic career. By the seventh trimester, it was my parents again who kindly helped me cover it. During that term, I married my best friend, a beautiful and cheerful Puerto Rican that I knew from my first day in chiropractic school. We studied together every day, and connected as we learned and grew up together in a foreign country to ours.

I remember how easy it was to get married. We were close to a court, so we asked ourselves, "What do we need to get married?". We went into court and asked. The judge asked us: "Are you of legal age? Do you have identification? You can get married right now. The ceremony can be this next Saturday, but you can sign today."

It was easy to do, because we knew our lives had to be lived together. I couldn't imagine being far from my cheerful Puerto Rican. We got married just like that and, two weeks later, we had a beautiful and meaningful church ceremony. My husband started the process for my US permanent residence, and in less than three months I was already a US resident. Thus, I was able to pay my last five quarters with my federal student loans, since I could have them as a resident.

I understand it was my faith in what we do not see, and the power to believe and see above the circumstances, that led me to where I am. My focus was on what I had to do, not how I would do it. I knew that something greater than my current situation guided my life. Today, my husband and I work together as chiropractors, and as he says: "we enjoy, we jump, and we laugh" daily, lovingly serving everyone who seeks our help to change their paradigm of life and health to make them whole.

Many times, we try to analyze everything, but our analytical mind cannot see the greatness of what may be possible on its own. Do not let your five senses fool you. Have faith, look with your heart and give yourself permission to do something extraordinary on this planet. Perhaps unconsciously you compare yourself with others and live in their shadows as an individual or professional; the collective perceptions around you limit you.

To create a better life and health, think beyond your current reality. **You cannot keep having the same thoughts and expect your life and health to change.** Your beliefs are what's most important for your progress, but they have to be aligned with your dreams. Keep the result you expect in mind, think about what it can be. By changing your thoughts, you will change your emotions, feelings, and behaviors. You will change the biology and chemistry in your body. You will change your reality. Have you noticed how people of great influence, who have inspired humanity, distinguish themselves by having thoughts greater than their current state?

When you are in a crisis or trauma situation, such as when you receive a bleak diagnosis, your focus is on what you do not want to happen rather than what you want to happen. This happens due to stress hormones. But, living in stress is just surviving, preparing for the worst that can happen. Be mindful in the present moment.

Focus on the result as if you already had it. Focus on what you want to happen, such as the healing of your body, instead of your fear of being sick.

I like how Wayne Dyer put it: our life is more like riding a boat than riding in a car. If you go in a car and turn the wheel, it responds immediately, but if you go in a boat, it is not like that. If you go on a boat and turn the wheel, what happens? NOTHING, until after a while. So your life is more like being on a boat. Anything you do is not necessarily going to give immediate results.

Changing thought patterns can take time and practice because they are deeply ingrained in your subconscious. You have created a habit, a strongly marked circuit in your brain. Start creating new circuits that help you create the optimal environment for your body and life to heal today.

I hope that you enrich your health and your life by having a healed mind, that you do not wait for something else to be diagnosed or for some trauma to arrive before you decide to make changes.

Brain and Heart in Harmony

Let me tell you a little about your heart. Personally, I am passionate about and attracted to learning about new scientific discoveries about the heart. In 1991, there was a discovery of nerve cells in the human heart. Your heart has approximately 40,000 specialized nerve cells, just like the cells in your brain[17]. You have neural cells in your heart that are arranged peculiarly. Scientists call these cells "the little brain in your heart"[18].

Your heart has intelligence. The heart's brain learns, remembers, feels, thinks, perceives, decides. This is real. It's not just a cute thing to read, it's literally true. There are many stories of people who received heart transplants, and their experiences receiving the new organ are fascinating. Many of them remember the life experiences of the person who donated their heart.

Scientific experts at the Institute of *HeartMath* can measure the energy of your heart and brain, and they know that when they are working in harmony, you optimize the healing power in you[19]. Your body was designed to optimally self-regulate by harmonizing the heart and brain.

The Institute of *HeartMath* continues to study the power of the heart[20]. The electromagnetic field generated by the heart is the strongest that your body produces. An electromagnetic field is a field generated by electric charges. It is reported at the speed of light, and, in fact, we can identify it as light. Your body produces electrical currents because of the chemical reactions of the different functions of the body.

We live surrounded by electric fields everywhere, but they are invisible to the human eye. Your body is energy, and it surrounds you. The energy of the heart is particularly important, since it is the strongest that your body generates. Energy from the heart enters and deepens into every cell in your body, and it can act as a synchronizing signal for all cells in your body analogously to the information carried by radio waves. Even other people can detect the energy of your heart and receive very important physiological effects.

The electromagnetic field of the heart is best organized during states of positive emotions. This is called coherence of the heart. Emotions like love, compassion, and appreciation are associated with an improved cardiac rhythm and reflect a greater synchronization in your nervous system. Researchers at the Institute of *HeartMath* established that by creating coherence in your heart and mind, you create 0.1 hertz between those two organs. On the other hand, when emotions are negative, such as anxiety, anger, or fear, the rhythm of your heart is less prominent and less synchronized with the nervous system.

As you can see, the greatness of the heart has no limits. Its energy can unite and synchronize all the cells in the body. Visualize the heart as the access point, the door in your body through which the energy of higher dimensional structures connects with the physical body[21]. I see it as the divine energy that gives life, using your heart as the door to reach all other cells and organs.

There are several extremely interesting studies that speak of the power of the energy emitted by the heart and the intention of your mind on the DNA molecule. I'll share one study I find very relevant to the mind and heart working in harmony and its effect on the body[22]. The study comprised putting DNA samples into test tubes. They asked each participant in the group to take a test in three different ways for approximately two minutes each.

1. They instructed each participant in the first group to generate a heart-focused state of mind (generating feelings of love and appreciation) while holding a clear intention to cause a specific change in DNA.

2. They instructed each participant in the second group to be in a heart-focused state of mind (generating feelings of love and appreciation) but without intending to change DNA.

3. They instructed each participant in the third group to be in a neutral state of emotions, but with the intention of causing a specific change in DNA.

They measured each individual's DNA makeup before and after each test. They calculated results based on the percentage of change from the baseline at the beginning of each trial. The really significant change in the DNA molecules occurred when the participants generated coherent feelings of the heart and had the intention to change the structure of the DNA; In those cases, up to 25% change could be measured, while in the other two tests there was no significant change (approximately a little over 1%).

In other words, when mind and heart are in harmony, they create results. Thoughts + healthy emotions = results.

The way my youngest son understood this concept was: the brain is king, and the heart is queen.

You raise your energy when your mind and heart work in tandem, when you align your thoughts with your emotions. You impact the physical world when your thoughts have a direct relationship with what you are feeling. So when people deliberately thought about the DNA change and also felt as if it had already happened, the miracle happened.

Since the 1900s, Max Planck, the father of quantum physics, discovered that humans have a quantum brain, which can create changes and transform matter. Your **thoughts** generate an electric field that activates the circumstances that are already available to you, and your **emotions** create the magnetism for you to make them come true in your life. So align your thoughts with your emotions to create what you seek. Create a harmony between mind and heart.

In the quantum field of all possibilities, states of health, well-being, fulfillment, abundance, success, love and compassion all already exist. What you need is to connect with this field by having your mind and heart in harmony. The universe understands vibrations. You will interact with it when your electromagnetic vibration, thoughts, and emotions are coherent with that field.

So, you cannot expect health and abundance to come into your life if you are not in vibrational agreement with what you long for. Realize that you live in a universe where everything can happen, where all the conditions are already in place to achieve what you are looking for.

There is a quantum level at which you are already healthy and where you are completely fulfilled in every area of your life, enjoying what you most want and yearn for. That reality already exists within the quantum field. You connect with this field by raising your energy or vibratory level to make it your new reality, but it already exists. Every thought and emotion that you generate is energy that brings you closer to or away from your new reality, optimal health, and the abundant life that you dream of having.

Masaru Emoto, Japanese author and researcher, wrote a fascinating book called *The Hidden Messages in Water* where he explains the results of his studies after investigating the impact that water molecules receive when they are in contact with thoughts and emotions, both positive and negative. He showed how the molecular structure of water responds to human conscious-ness. You can find amazing photos of his studies. For example, water molecules before a Mozart symphony get a much more uniform structure than water molecules before heavy metal mu-sic.

The water molecule changes, harmonizes and is much more beautiful when it is in the presence of messages of love, peace and gratitude. On the contrary, that molecule becomes cloudy and loses its brilliance when it is in the presence of negative messages, such as "you disturb me" or "you disgust me." If our body is 70-80% water, imagine how receptive we are to positive and negative thoughts and emotions.

It is vital that you have thoughts and can generate feelings of love and gratitude towards your body, towards each of your cells. Your body listens to you. Commonly, I instruct my patients to use phrases like: "I give love to my body; I give it permission to heal". At first I saw their surprised faces, but then they unders-tood and their smiling looks told me they recognize this truth.

When your mind and heart are in harmony, your body can generate around 1,300 positive biochemical reactions and has an optimal internal environment for healing. One of the biggest benefits to your health is the positive changes in your DNA[23]. More and more studies are showing how your DNA changes by doing these practices and how it prevents telomeres, which are the final and crucial part of the chromosome that acts to protect and ensure DNA replication, from breaking.

Another great benefit of having your brain and heart in harmony is the affinity you foster with your intuition, the inner voice that you have, which guides you to make decisions and to stay in balance. What we call "hunches" are messages from your heart. Let your heart speak to your mind.

When you connect with the guidance of your heart, your perception improves, as does your memory and the ability to learn new things. There is enormous power in your heart, a constant intelligence speaking to you. Everything that surrounds us is full of magical things, patiently waiting to be discovered when our senses become better tuned.

Indigenous people have long used techniques to harmonize the mind with the heart[24]. Also, we see this practice in the military with high performance athletes and intelligence agents, as they optimize their nervous system. When you live in harmony with your heart, you make a difference with everything around you.

Live moment by moment, within the heart's high frequency. This is the frequency where you can manifest, because you can communicate with your subconscious, which is the instrument of manifestation. Recognize that everything is moving in divine order, everything is connecting perfectly.

In the following lines, I briefly share a guide to harmonize your mind with your heart that I learned from the renowned author and scientist, Gregg Braden. Read first so you understand, and then put it into practice. You do not need music, you can play it, but it is unnecessary in order to harmonize your mind with your heart.

Guide to Harmonizing the Mind With the Heart

- Take slow, deep breaths for a minute. Just by breathing in this way, you tell your body that it is safe; you create an internal environment of healing for your body; you go from being in a sympathetic state to a para-sympathetic state in your nervous system. Your brain releases the chemistry necessary to heal everything that needs to heal and to rejuvenate. Stress hormones decline, as do inflammatory agents. Your immune system optimizes. There are immediate changes that can be detected in your saliva through the increase of secretory immunoglobulin A (SIgA), which is an antibody.

- Look at the center of your being. Imagine that you breathe deep into your heart.

- Touch your heart with your hand and allow your consciousness to pass from your mind to your heart. This is powerful. Here you tell your mind to be quiet, and to focus on your heart.

- Bring into your body a feeling of appreciation, love, gratitude, compassion, and caring. Notice the frequency of love reverberating in your body. This is a powerful way to communicate with your body.

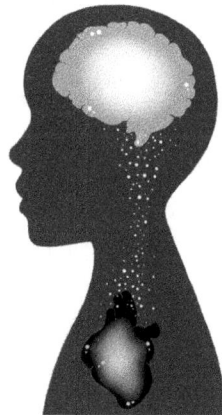

You can do this exercise every day. It should take at least three minutes. You are preparing your mind and your heart for your day. It's like when you go to the gym to exercise your body; by doing this exercise, you are exercising your mind and heart for whatever comes your way during the day, and filling your body with vitality.

It helps me greatly to harmonize my mind with my heart before I adjust my patients, as well as before a meeting or event, such as presenting a topic in public. It is like tuning an instrument; the brain gets in tune with the heart so that your body benefits as well as the people around you.

I hope you appreciate your body every day, that you build confidence in it. Have genuine compassion for yourself. Recognize that your physical body is made up of conscious cells that listen to your thoughts and perceive your emotions. Your body loves that you pay attention to it. Align your thinking with your emotions to create an inner environment of healing. You will bring a healing chemistry to your body. Live from your heart, don't be afraid to let go, trust and love. You will understand at last that love heals.

Beyond Genetics

From a very young age, I was taught that genetics determine our health and life. It was and still is the belief that the human being is a victim of his inheritance; for example, if my grandfather had heart disease, then that means that I also have the genetics to suffer from a heart condition, so I would expect to have the same disease as my grandfather.

However, the new biology teaches us that this is not the case. This is what epigenetics is about, (epi means above or beyond); **your health does not depend on genetics**. Maybe you learned you cannot control your biology, that in a way your future is already predetermined based on your genetics. Let me ask you, how do you respond if you think that the power to create your health is not in you? You give your power to something external, to what you consider to have the power to heal you.

My intention is to help you understand a little better how your cells work, as it will make it easier for you to understand how your body can heal. Every day, your body loses hundreds of billions of cells. Cells have their life cycles, and then they die to be replaced by other new cells. This is a normal and vital process for your body to have a state of homeostasis. Stem cells are always waiting for your body's signal to replace any type of cell. They can replace cells of the brain, muscles, bones, pancreas, intestines, and so on.

The renowned biologist, Bruce Lipton, who inspires me greatly, has devoted much of his life to the study of the cell, and what he has found is truly amazing. We can understand that what determines the future of cells is the environment in which they grow, not genetics. This has revolutionized biology, as it differs greatly from what we believed: it is not the genes that determine the future of the cell but the environment in which it is found.

Your body is a large collection of cells and microorganisms. Looking at yourself, you might think that you are a single entity, but in reality, your body is a large community of cells and microorganisms. The environment where your cells live is your blood. The conditions

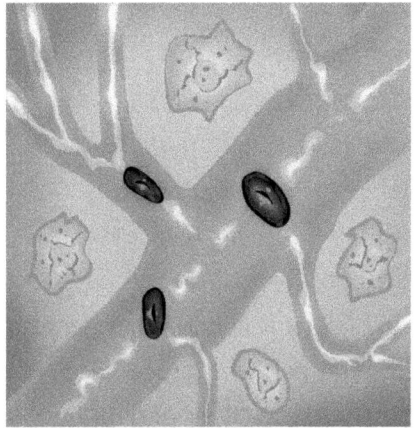

of the environment of your blood determine the future of your cells and the genetic response. In other words, your genes follow the order according to the environment of the cell. Your brain, the great conductor of the body, determines what chemicals your blood will have. And that determination is made according to the perception of your mind.

You change the chemistry in your blood by changing the perspective of your mind. Your brain translates your mind's perception into the chemistry your body will use. For example, your perception of love, compassion, and cooperation generates oxytocin, dopamine, and growth hormone. This is the chemistry that supports the vitality and growth of your cells.

If your mind perceives fear, your brain translates the perception of fear into a chemistry for your blood very differently; It will include stress hormones like cortisol and inflammatory agents. This is the chemistry to protect and survive, not to grow.

The cell membrane (the outer part of the cell) acts as the brain of the cell. It has receptors to obtain signals from the cell's external and internal environments and convert the information it gets into the biology necessary to keep the cell alive. The concept that genes control biology is wrong. Your genes behave according to the signals that the cell membrane receives around the environment. Your genes wait for the signal of how and when to activate.

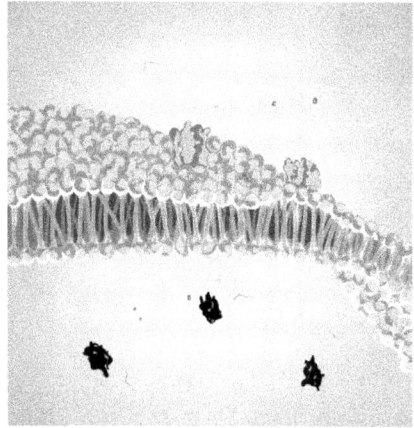

Have you heard of spontaneous remission? If you do some research, you'll encounter the multitude of stories from around the world regarding this subject. Spontaneous remission is when people instantly heal illnesses in ways that doctors do not explain, because they are not medically possible. Spontaneous remission is the beautiful result of a true perspective transformation. Change of perspective means change in the chemistry that your brain generates for the environment of the cells in your body.

The power to heal is in the consciousness and not in the person's genetics. Your biology will agree with your state of consciousness. This new biology of epigenetics empowers you, because you can change your belief from being a victim of your genetics to being a creator of the expression of your genes.

From Wanting to Achieving

You might question yourself and think that it is not so easy to heal just by changing your perspective, and I agree in part, because you have deep-seated subconscious thoughts that you can reprogram to support your conscious mind.

Your mind is divided into two parts: subconscious and conscious. I remind you that the subconscious mind is instincts and habits, which you do automatically, and it makes up approximately 95% of your actions. It is the primordial programming that was formed in your mind from before you were born to approximately seven years of age. It does not come from your personal yearnings; it was formed from observing others, such as your parents, your siblings, teachers, and so on. In this way, you got behaviors copied from others, which do not indicate your true desires but the programs you learned as a child.

Your conscious mind is the part that creates, aspires, wants, and longs. It is the part that wants to heal and be well. Maybe your subconscious does not have the proper programming to support your conscious. If, as a child, you were taught the lack of power and limitations, those are programs you took from others and not from yourself. For this reason, you struggle to externalize what your conscious wants.

Subconscious Mind	Conscious Mind
Instincts	The part that wants to heal
Habits (past)	Present time
What you do automatically	Pays attention to details
95% of your actions	5% of your conduct and decisions
Primary programming (before being born until approximately seven years old)	Intelectual intelligence
Formed by observing others	Rational
Copied conduct	Creator
Does not come from your personal longings	Shows your true desires
Does not highlight your true desires	Your true aspirations
Comfortable and familiar	Unknown and possible

Recognizing your subconscious programming is the first step; It gives you the opportunity to change habits of thinking and acting that do not align with your true desires, and thus you can change your health and your life. Eliminating limiting programs you learned as a child can take practice. You may not change your schedule overnight, but you will succeed if it is your genuine intention to do so.

You can rewrite your subconscious programming with programs that support your conscious longings, free you from disease, and help you live a fuller life. Many times, your subconscious associates with your comfortable areas, with what you already know. It wants to stay within your habits and what's normal to you.

These are some practical tips that can help you in reprogramming your subconscious. Review them as much as necessary until they become part of you.

- Befriend change. Let life flow through you. Discover the power and great opportunity that lie in the unknown. Open your mind and your heart so that you see you are guided, and that everything fits perfectly. Be willing to see what is possible. You will only see miracles when you actually expect to see them.

- Give yourself permission to recognize the abundance that is in you and in everything around you. Think that you are part of it and it is part of you. "You are not a drop in the ocean. You are the entire ocean, in a drop."- Rumi. Abundance surrounds you and you can see it on all sides, just like the endless sky with its beautiful contrast of colors. The flowers where you walk, the green grass, the plants, the birds in the trees are all results of abundance. Also, look at the abundance of your body, with trillions of cells and microorganisms. Know that this world of abundance was created for you. The limit is determined by your thinking. Look at yourself, recognize that you are the highest and most perfect creation of your Creator and that the abundance you see is available to you. You can vibrate higher by recognizing that if something is on your mind, you can shape it. Build in your mind the life you want to have. You can shape it. There is abundance in every aspect of your life. What defines each person comes from their state of consciousness. You are a spiritual being, always expanding, always growing. Have this concept of abundance in your subconscious. You are an abundant being in every aspect of your life and in every cell of your body. Open your mind and heart to the good, as it is your right at birth. The abundance that you can see in others is available to you. It is real, it is not a fantasy. Recognize the abundance that is in you and in everything around you.

• Surround yourself with positive and constructive support. Make sure the areas you frequent offer you that ongoing support. In your office, your home, and even in the car, keep taped messages of key phrases that help you reprogram your subconscious. The more you see them, the more they will be a part of your new subconscious. Listen to affirmations and inspirations from early in the morning and before going to sleep, since in those hours your brain is in theta waves, which are what help you reprogram your subconscious. Remember, your subconscious was formed during your childhood, when theta waves were the ones that ruled your brain as a child. Surround yourself with people who give you support and inspiration. I recognize the great value that my mentors have brought to my life, both personally and professionally. At certain times, we need someone who can broaden our vision. We live in a world of cooperation, and being open to the support that others can offer is a great virtue. You can also enrich other lives. "We rise by lifting others up." - Robert Ingersoll.

- Talk about what you want to achieve as something existing in the present, grateful for it as if you already have it. Create in the present moment the experience in your heart of having what you want. Keep those powerful feelings alive, the ones that will produce everything you wish for; the strength to create flows from your heart. This is how prayer works: we do not get what we ask for, but through faith and the lack of doubt, we believe that everything we need already exists in our life (Matthew 21: 21-22 and Mark 11:24). Change your perspective on the world. By asking for something, we unconsciously affirm that we do not have what we are looking for. The bridge between us and what we long for is faith, a feeling of full belief in our heart. These are quantum principles that apply to spirituality. That is why I mention we are living in a time where science and spirituality come together. You can perceive your prayer as something that already has an answer, feel it already existing. It will bring you to your inner place of joy, the place that produces tears of happiness. For example, when praying for rain, enjoy and appreciate how water feels on your body, smell the scent of wet earth, and give thanks for it. "Therefore, I tell you that whatever you ask for while praying, believe that you will receive it, and it will come to you" - Mark 11:24 (KJV 1960). "You will doubt, not only will you do this of the fig tree, but if you say to this mountain: Take off and throw yourself into the sea, it will be done. And whatever you ask in prayer, believing, you will receive"- Matthew 21: 21-22 (RVR 1960).

- Create a space to visualize the type of legacy you want to leave. Keep in mind the big picture of your heart's desire. What would you be doing right now if you had all the time and money in the world? Your job is to know what you have to do; your Creator will handle the "how".

- Identify what your limiting thoughts are. Some may be hidden because something ingrained them in your subconscious from a very young age. Identify them so that you can change them.

- Get in the habit of writing reasons you are grateful for everyday. You can keep a journal by your bedside. This will make your mind aware of what you already have rather than what you need. Nothing will bring you as much abundance in every area of your life as gratitude.

CONSTRUCT #4:

Divine Nourishment at Your Pace

Does Your Lifestyle Support Your Health?

Nourishing yourself the way your Creator designed for your body is what I call *divine nourishment*. Humanity used to eat what the Earth gave us; now we eat what the food industry produces. The processed food industry began in 1910 after the invention of trans fats. By 1940, it had grown dramatically, and we are now seeing the health results of this type of diet.

No matter what your diet has been in the past, the most important time for you is now, because that is where your power to decide and create changes lies. Raising your consciousness in the present makes you make your decisions from your essence. Your power begins with knowing who you are and what it means to nurture your body consciously. The recommendations that I share with you in this chapter are part of a lifestyle that supports your health. They are based on a vitalistic vision, which recognizes the innate intelligence within the body.

As a society, we have forgotten where we came from. When you were born, you arrived on a planet that has everything you need to nourish your body: all the food on Earth, fresh and full of nutrients, gives life to your body. It could not be any other way. You were created in love, on a planet of love, where everything you need has been provided for you.

We cannot expect to have life in our body if we only feed it with lifeless food. See nature as the source of your food. Recognize and adopt in your lifestyle the foods that have life and minimize the processed stuff. This way, you will maintain balance, variety, and moderation through divine nourishment.

Ingest the Food That Nature Designed for You

Observing nature always helps us understand everything better. Let its peace teach you; take the time to contemplate the details that surround you, because returning to nature is returning to your origin here on Earth. Learning from it and taking care of it gives you life. Focus on all food that comes from the Earth because it has life and, therefore, it gives you sustenance.

When you ask yourself what to eat, ask these questions also: where did that food come from: from a tree, plant, root, seed? Did it come from your Creator? If you consume meat or animal products, ask yourself: what did that animal eat and how was it raised? For example, the chicken eggs you had for breakfast this morning, did they come from happy hens that roam freely, saw the sun and fed on the earth, or, on the contrary, did they live locked up and full of stress without seeing the sunlight, and worse, their bodies full of hormones and antibiotics?

Once you raise your consciousness, it becomes easy to recognize the food that was designed for you. If we evaluate what the strongest animals on our planet eat, such as horses and gorillas, we see they obtain their nutrients directly from the Earth.

A single kick from a horse can knock a person down. Where do they get their bone strength? It comes from the nutrients in the plants they eat and not from other animal or dairy products, which you might think are necessary for strong, healthy bones.

Eat what was designed for you to eat, what nature offers you.

The human being wants to taste and eat as much as possible. Isn't it amazing that the little moisture-wicking packets you find in your new shoe box or new purse clearly say "not for human consumption"? Most likely, we would want to try it if those words were not so explicit.

Adapting to food that is closer to nature, cleaner and fresher, can take time, because since childhood, society programs you to eat in a certain way. Start with the foods you already know and gradually try new, fresh foods. Open your mind and palate to new flavors. Below, I share a table with some of the most nutritious foods, classified by the nutrients they offer and their main functions.

Seven Super Foods

(content from https://www.mercola.com/infographics/superfoods.htm)

Super Food	Content	Some of Their Functions
Spirulina	Chlorophyll (oxygen), amino acids: 65% - 71% complete protein, which represents 22% more protein than beef; variety of vitamins and minerals: vitamin A, E, D, B1, B3, B6, B12, iron, zinc, folic acid, essential fatty acids, nucleic acids, numerous antioxidants.	Protects your cardiovascular system, lowers the risk of cancer, keeps your blood pressure and cholesterol at optimal levels, supports the growth of good bacteria in your stomach, helps fight Candida infections, provides support for allergies.
Chlorella	Gamma-Aminobutyric Acid (GABA), Iron, Vitamin B12, Folate, Complete Amino Acids.	Helps improve insulin sensitivity, normalizes blood pressure and sugar levels, increases energy levels, helps with your ability to concentrate and focus, supports the elimination of toxins including metals such as mercury.
Brussels sprouts	Magnesium, phosphorus, vitamins A, K, C, B 6, B12, thiamine, potassium, folate, copper, manganese, iron, calcium, high amount of fiber.	Supports your immune system, pro-duces enzymes that help cleanse your body of toxins that cause cancer, helps fight diseases by having detoxi-fying properties, promotes healthy DNA, its potassium content helps the heart and blood pressure, assists in the strength of your bones.
Kale	Antioxidants lutein and zeaxanthin, vitamins A, B and C, calcium, fiber, iron, chlorophyll, nature-3-carbinol, 9 essential amino acids, omega 3.	Helps your stomach, liver and immune system, benefits the respiratory system, protects against cancer, helps improve cholesterol levels.
Broccoli	Vitamin C, E, flavonoids quercetin and kaemferol, beta carotenes, lutein, sulfurophane, vitamin K, folate, calcium, fiber.	Helps your digestive system, promotes detoxification, supports your body to avoid or fight cancer, hypertension, allergies, diabetes, osteoarthritis.
Artichoke	Vitamin C, K, magnesium, manganese, copper, potassium, phosphorus, fiber, antioxidants, and phytonutrients such as quercetin, rutin, gallic acid, and cynarin.	Supports the digestive system and liver, helps normalize cholesterol and triglyceride levels.
Açaí Berry	Antioxidants, anthocyanins, iron, calcium, vitamin A, amino acids.	Supports your immune system, provides anti-aging benefits, helps improve your energy, destroys cancer cells.

Leaving your food comfort zones can bring big and positive changes to your health. Think of it as a learning path rather than a fight for power. Have feelings of love and compassion for yourself, and always be grateful for the new opportunities that each day brings you. If you have children, be flexible when making changes to make the process positive and sustainable.

Children learn from what they see. They have to watch Mom or Dad eat consciously and healthily so they can do the same. Remember that their subconscious is formed by looking at you. Involve your children in preparing the menu and meals whenever possible. You can allow them to choose their snacks. Surround yourself with people who are on the same path as you and share recipes with them.

I take this opportunity to share with you a beautiful experience we had in our practice. The mission in our office is "to love, educate and adjust every patient who seeks our help." The education part is vital for our patients, and every month we give educational workshops. One favorite is the recipe workshop. In it, patients choose a healthy recipe, full of valuable nutrients, and prepare it at home to bring it to the event.

We very much enjoy watching communities develop and bond through sharing healthy meals and recipes. Everyone recognizes they are not the only ones seeking health. The food is always exquisite and has the power to unite. It may surprise you to see that you have many people around you who are quietly changing their diet.

To nurture your inspiration, you can follow chefs cooking with a focus on raw and sustainable foods on social media, where the vision is to include a variety of plants, legumes, vegetables, greens, fruits, seeds, and nuts. Sustainable change can take time to happen. **Remember that it is not a diet, it is a healthy eating style that supports the functions of your body.**

What materials do you want to build your house from? I imagine you want the best quality ones. Your body is your first home, so opt for the best quality food (materials) to build it. Recognize that what you had for breakfast today or what you had for lunch or dinner is being converted, thanks to the innate intelligence of your body, into cells of the pancreas, heart, liver, skin, etc. You decide every day the quality with which you will create your home.

What is the best nutrition for you? Maybe you struggle to know exactly what to eat. I propose that you to listen to your body, be aware of what helps and benefits it. Eventually, you realize that the best food is one that brings you closer to nature.

There are many food-related classifications nowadays, so many that they could confuse you. There are also a lot of names for different ways of eating. Learn to listen to your body and you will see that you can discern which is the best. Always remember that whatever you choose, the driving force should always be to consume food that comes from nature. Some classifications of different ways of eating are:

- Vegan - omit all types of animal products, including eggs, dairy, honey, or gelatin.
- Vegetarian - skip meat and seafood but consume dairy and other animal products, such as honey.
- Flexitarian - eat mostly a vegetarian diet but eat meat occasionally.
- Pegan - focuses on eating vegetables, fruits, nuts, seeds, meat, fish, and eggs while avoiding dairy, legumes, grains, sugar, and processed foods.

- Plant-based diet - consumes plant-derived foods such as vegetables, grains, seeds, legumes, and fruits, with little or no animal products.
- Raw-vegan - consumes food that comes from the Earth and is in its natural state, strictly organic and vegetable, and completely omits the consumption of any meat or derivative of animal origin.
- Pescetarian - focuses on eating fish, shellfish, and other forms of animal products such as dairy, but does not eat chicken, beef, and pork.
- Keto - low in carbohydrates, high in good fats and proteins of animal or vegetable origin.
- Paleo - focuses on clean meats, fish, fruits, vegetables, nuts and seeds, avoiding dairy, legumes and grains as well as everything processed.

The way you eat also depends on where you live. For example, Inuits in northern Alaska, Canada, and Greenland eat a diet low in carbohydrates but high in fat and protein. They are an example of a population with very low levels of atherosclerosis, hypertension and even dental caries compared to more westernized populations.

Another great example is the population of Okinawa in Japan, a country with a higher life expectancy and more centenarians than others. When you observe that culture, you realize they eat seasonal foods and choose to let nature set the pace, and not resort to vegetables from other places or forced cultivation in greenhouses. In this way, they do not alter the nature of food; they eat what nature gives them. In general, the Japanese diet has a high rate of carbohydrates found in vegetables, fruits, and whole grains, such as rice. Their fishmongers and butchers offer fresh products.

I encourage you to eat consciously and take note of how your body responds to the foods you eat. Observe how much or how little energy they provide you. Analyze your body's sensations after eating what you have ingested and determine if there is any pain in any part of your body, such as a headache, pain in your hands, inflammation in your stomach. You will find eventually that your body wants you to seek food from the Earth, fresh and clean. By consciously listening to your body, you will learn to discern what is best for you.

The Three Errors of Modern Nutrition

Today, much of the modern diet consists of processed food, a lot of which contain the three biggest dangers of modern eating: chemicals, sugars, and bad fats.

1) Chemicals - Choose What Is the Least Toxic

We are exposed to toxins or chemicals every day. In fact, your body produces its own toxins or waste as a result of all its functions. These toxins are known as endogenous wastes (carbon dioxide, ammonia, and free radicals).

Your body innately knows how to flush out toxins and cleanse itself..

You may consider that there is not much you can do to control the chemicals or toxins produced outside of your body (exogenous toxins), which are found in medicines and vaccines, processed food, the air you breathe, the water you drink, or the products you use[25]. **It is entirely possible to live drug-free by living a healthy lifestyle that recognizes the health and life builders discussed in this book.** It will always be in your power to choose the least harmful, natural, local and seasonal foods and products.

An overload of chemicals or external toxins can interfere with your body's innate ability to cleanse or detoxify itself and lead to a state of illness.

Una sobrecarga de químicos o toxinas externas puede interferir con la habilidad innata de tu cuerpo de limpiarse o detoxificarse a sí mismo y llevarlo a un estado de enfermedad.

The statistics in the United States are very shocking. For example, we use more than 800 million pounds of herbicides each year[26]. We can find over 160 industrial chemicals in the average adult body[27]. There are approximately 80,000 chemicals registered for every day use[28]. Some signs of high levels of chemicals or toxicity in your body can be joint pain, skin problems, constipation, tiredness, difficulty sleeping, headache, sinusitis, difficulty concentrating and irritability, among other things. All these are signals that your body gives you to warn you: it warns you, it warns you, and it continues to warn you. Listen to it, otherwise the amount of toxicity in your body can make your body seriously ill.

Aim to avoid foods that come with hormones, vaccines, pesticides, fertilizers, antibiotics, and chemical additives, as well as all kinds of artificial and diet sweeteners, as these are highly carcinogenic and inflammatory. Another goal is to eliminate transgenic or genetically modified foods, better known as Genetically Modified Organisms (GMOs). These are foods in which the genetic material was artificially manipulated, most times in a laboratory through genetic engineering.

More and more countries are notifying the consumer about which foods are free of genetic material and you can read it on the labels reading *non-GMO* and *organic*. If you decide to switch to an organic diet and eat meat, I recommend starting with the animal products, as the chemicals in ordinary meat can "bio-magnify" in your body. For this reason, try to get the meat you source from animals that have been fed and raised free of chemicals.

I want to clarify that it is unnecessary to eat meat to get the amount of daily protein necessary for the proper functioning of your body. You can always get protein from a plant source. Here are some examples of foods high in protein: kidney beans, legumes such as chickpeas and lentils, quinoa, amaranth, rye, wild or basmati rice, oats, walnuts, peanuts, almonds, wheat germ, avocado, coconut, spinach, spirulina, watercress, sweet potato or yams, seeds such as pumpkin, sesame, hemp, sesame, sunflower, chia, edamame, peas, tempeh and tofu, among others.

You might find it costly to eat healthy or chemical-free, but it all depends on your perspective and priorities. We all spend on what we consider a priority. Do you know how much cancer treatment costs? Do you have any idea what a dialysis session costs? Think that, by eating consciously, you are investing in your health and then not having to invest in your disease. **Taking care of your health will never be more expensive than taking care of yourself during illness.**

I remember once standing in line at a supermarket when, suddenly, the lady in front of me looked closely at my shopping cart and then said to me: "wow, that's going to be expensive!" I looked at her with a smile and amiably replied: "This represents my family's and my health plan. What I invest here, I save on medications and hospitalizations." From there, we continued our conversation, and to this day, she is one of the most loyal patients in our office.

If you have the time, you can create your own organic garden at home; it would be ideal for you and your family. Imagine eating from your own garden and inspiring your children or grandchildren to do the same. You can also support local farmers' markets that can give you the assurance that they produced the food they offer sustainably.

2) What is Not So Sweet About Sugar

Sugar is a generic term for simple carbohydrates. It is in almost everything processed. You find it in mayonnaise, ketchup, breads, cereals, juices, sodas, candy, baby food, refined cereals, and the list goes on.

Consuming sugar is highly addictive and toxic to the body.

Sugar has the ability to weaken your immune system almost immediately after consumption, negatively impacting your energy levels[29]. Sugar creates inflammation in your body[30]. It is the main food cause for pathogens and cancer cells[31]. It is associated with higher levels of depression in both men and women[32],[33].

Another important effect on your body is how it impacts you cells telomeres, since sugar makes them shorter reducing your cells functions[34]. Telomeres are the cells protective shield, a compound structure at the end of the chromosome that shortens over the years when cells divide to multiply and regenerate tissues and organs.

The food industry has many names for different sugars. The one that I most urge you to avoid is corn syrup, also known as high fructose corn syrup, since it is highly toxic. Unfortunately, it is added to the vast majority of processed foods. To sweeten your food or drinks, I suggest you use coconut sugar, whole stevia leaf powder or liquid, monk fruit sugar, also known as *Luo Han Guo*, agave, honey, or dried fruits such as ripe bananas or dates.

Refined bread and white rice quickly turn to sugar. If you consume breads, try to purchase the artisan kind that is free of processed flours, chemicals and added sugars. For example, you can choose a rye, millet, cassava, kamut, yucca or spelt bread.

Swap white rice for brown, basmati, jasmine, or wild rice, or millet, quinoa, and couscous. Modify the refined cereal with whole grains such as wheat germ, oats, barley, millet, quinoa, amaranth, kamut and saracene. Swap white flours for less processed whole wheat flours and pasta such as cassava, almond, pumpkin, chickpea, coconut, and quinoa.

You will learn that there is always a healthy alternative to what you usually eat. It is all a matter of finding the least processed foods that are closer to nature. You will find a multitude of nutrients and beneficial properties for your health.

3) Fats - Avoid the Bad Kinds and Increase the Healthy Ones

Fats are an essential part of your nourishment and of vital importance to your body. To give you an idea of its importance, your body's cells have a cell membrane made up of fats, and it is 50% of its weight[35]. This membrane facilitates communication between the cells, their movement and fluidity, the selective permeability of the molecules they pass through, and the transduction of signals.

60% of your brain is fat, and to maintain optimal brain function, you need high-quality fatty acids (omega-3 and omega-6), along with antioxidants that protect them from oxidation. Your body cannot live without good fats, which is why it's important to find foods that provide healthy fats.

Go back to whole foods that provide good fats. For example, wild or deep-sea fish that are not farm-raised and nuts and seeds like chia and hemp. If you want avocado oil, use the avocado itself. You can use flax seeds instead of flaxseed oil. If you want sesame seed oil, use sesame seeds, walnuts, dried fruit, or organic (cold-pressed) coconut oil.

For cooking, use grape seed oil, which has a very high nutritional power, rich in proteins, minerals, vitamins and antioxidants. It is also the most resistant to high temperatures, and this makes it the best for cooking. Good fats or essential oils are polyunsaturated fats, necessary for the different functions of your nervous system, such as good memory, emotional balance, social adaptations, attention, learning, mental agility and prevention of brain aging.

It is vitally important to incorporate good fats from childhood, since this is when the brain is forming the quickest.

However, not all fats benefit you. Those found in vegetable oils, which predominate in processed and fried foods, fast foods and industrial pastries, are known as transgenic or "trans" fats[36]. Transgenic fat was the first processed food that entered the food industry in 1910. In its manufacturing process, hydrogen is added to vegetable oil in order to increase the preservation time of processed food and to preserve its flavor.

Trans fats react with oxygen and create free radicals during metabolism[37]. When the body has a high amount of free radicals and antioxidants are not enough to counteract their effects, oxidative stress occurs, the great producer of the chronic diseases that we know today. Oxidative stress changes the structure and function of the cell, which is why it favors different diseases. This shuts down your immune system.

Some of the most common diseases related to trans fats are cardiovascular diseases, cancer, diabetes, allergies, obesity, and neurological conditions. Counteracting the action of free radicals is possible if you provide your body with the necessary antioxidants found in vitamins, minerals and enzymes that the body synthesizes from a healthy diet. Your goal is to seek food closer to its natural state or, as I see it, its divine state.

Another unfavorable factor of processed foods is that they hinder the body's satisfaction process. In July 2019, the Cell Metabolism Journal published a study[38] on how processed food slows down your body's satisfaction process, making you eat larger amounts.

They divided the group of twenty participants into two: ten of them were given highly processed meals, while they gave the other ten whole and unprocessed foods. The foods contained the same amount of calories, carbohydrates, protein, fat, and fiber. They encouraged the participants to eat until they were satisfied.

The results showed that those who ate processed foods ate an average of 508 more calories a day. In just two weeks, participants who ate the processed food gained an average of one kilogram, while those who ate unprocessed foods lost one kilogram.

Much of the processed food is deficient in many nutrients, which can stimulate more consumption. The study also showed a big difference in hormonal values. People who ate fresh unprocessed foods showed higher levels of the peptide hormone YY (PYY), which suppresses the appetite, as well as lower levels of ghrelin, the hunger-inducing hormone.

In contrast, the group of people who ate processed food showed lower levels of the appetite-suppressing hormones (PYY) and higher levels of the appetite-creating hormones (ghrelin). The group that ate processed foods ate more quickly. Processed food is easier to eat, as it is softer and easier to chew. Signs of satiety arrive approximately fifteen to twenty minutes after being satiated. For this reason, it is important to eat food slowly.

Conscious Consumption for Your Day to Day

Healthy eating does not depend only on what you put on your plate or what you prepare in your kitchen. It has a lot to do with your consciousness, with the perception of your mind.

Seek balance. Balance yourself between overindulging and depriving yourself when eating. Pay attention to your body and be aware of when you are hungry and when you are not. Every day is different, and your body has different physiological needs; you don't have to eat the same portions every day.

You do not have to eat just because it is mealtime. Feed your body until your innate intelligence lets you know that you are satisfied and not until you finish the plate. Take your time supplying food to your body. It should not be all at once, nor a large quantity all at once.

Your digestive system is like a campfire, where combustion increases if you add wood slowly and dies down if you add a lot of wood in one go. Likewise, you digest in a better way when you eat little by little. Eat calmly, savor and enjoy every bite you take. What you eat and how you eat is important. **Stop when you consider that your hunger is satisfied. Remember that it takes your brain approximately fifteen to twenty minutes to pick up on your level of satiety.**

Do not hurt your body by unconsciously treating it like a garbage disposal because you feel pressured to finish your plate. Not wanting to throw away the excess, or consuming food from the fridge before it goes bad, does the same. The famous saying: "what does not kill you makes you stronger", is not very accurate. In reality, what does not kill you can take your life away gradually. What impacts your health and life the most are the little habits that you do daily.

Do not stop meals to lose weight, as you will create the opposite effect, because restlessness and suppressed hunger will motivate you to eat more than you need. Love yourself and respect your body. Be grateful for it every day.

Writing down what your biggest cravings are could help you control them: sweets, alcohol, cold cuts, ice cream, salty cravings, and so on. You can see that, most of the time, the reason you have such an exuberant attraction to a particular product is the association of food with day-to-day situations.

Inspect your connection to the attachment. Contemplate the habits that you resist letting go. Ask yourself if the results you get are productive or if it solves internal conditions such as anger, helplessness, anxiety and anguish.

Cravings often mask moods. At sixteen years old, a few months after leaving my home and my country, I had bulimia. I had episodes where I stopped eating for many hours, even a whole day, and then, when night came and I could not bear the hunger, I would devour everything I found.

The next morning, before the sun came up, I was ready with my tennis shoes on the track in the park near the house where I lived. Guilt for having eaten so much the night before made me run for hours and hours. I ran for three to four hours before getting ready to go to school. So much so that the neighbors thought I trained to run long-distance marathons.

Although I enjoyed seeing the results in the athletic condition of my legs and the stamina I gained, I carried an intense and constant internal fight. The biggest lesson was to recognize that I was drowning my emotions with food, as if it were literally a drug, to avoid my internal struggle in the middle of many life changes.

I missed my parents and family, my home country and its culture. At the same time, I recognized the great blessing I had of living abroad and having the possibilities to study in an incredibly healthy environment, with great people who marked my life for the better. I felt a different pain. I call it internal growth pain; I understood everything was part of something bigger in my life.

That experience taught me that there is strength in pausing, looking inward, and acknowledging those feelings as part of an important growth process. You can trust that life is on your side and wants to support the longings of your heart if you just believe enough. Clear up those emotional states and deal with them, put food aside, learn not to associate it with your emotional state by being present in your mind.

Dare to let go of old habits and create new ones that are more beneficial for you.

Determine what you want to create physically and emotionally. How healthy do you want to be? What kind of life do you want to live, sedentary or active? Visualize and program who you want to be. Your energy will go where your focus is. Avoid bad-mouthing people, especially while eating. Refrain from criticizing the way others eat, if they eat little or eat a lot, if they eat badly, because words are powerful.

Always be grateful for the energy in the food you eat, that becomes part of your body.

Practice consciousness when shopping, cooking, eating, and even washing dishes. Have you ever enjoyed washing dishes? You can! Feel the water in your hands, appreciate the sensations and movements of your hands and the objects you clean. You can be aware of every detail and thus bring enjoyment even to the simplest of your day activities.

The way you eat reflects yourself, and this manifests itself in everything you do. **Be fully aware that what you eat will become cells in your body, just as your experiences become part of your life.**

Always try to have a feeling of gratitude for everything that the planet and nature gives you, for the effort of those who work the soil and show you generosity when preparing your food, and for others when it is your turn to cook, choosing whole foods and eliminating chemicals whenever possible.

Enjoy your food. It was made to be enjoyed, and don't miss out on the experience of sharing it with others. Realize that each experience, although it may seem mundane and repetitive, is unique and unrepeatable.

CONSTRUCT #5:

Oxygenation in Water, and Movement

Water – What Creates Life

You have probably heard that your body is made up of 60% - 70% water, depending on your age. But have you really thought about what this fact means? Your body is more water than any other compound[39]. It is the main material of your cells, tissues and organs.

To make it a little clearer, approximately 73% of your brain and heart is water[40,41]. 90% of your plasma is water[42], 83% of your lungs is water, 64% of your skin is water, 79% of your kidneys and muscles is water, 31% of your bones is water[43]. Incredible right?

The most impressive thing for me is knowing that the water molecules in our body change according to our thoughts and feelings. Remember that famous study by Masaru Emoto, where he studied how thoughts and emotions impact the world around us? Water behaves differently depending on how you see it. See it as life-creating material, have a feeling of love and gratitude towards the water. Many countries have a cultural tradition where they do not drink water without thanking it first.

Knowing your body is approximately 60% - 70% water molecules and they change according to your thoughts and feelings, ask yourself: how is your body? Being aware of the power you have over your body is very important. Realize that you can design both your healing and your illness. **Your body works according to your instructions. Give your cells conscious instructions, give them permission to heal.**

Life Depends on Water

Water is not just a colorless, tasteless liquid. These are some of its vital benefits: it eliminates toxins, hydrates organs, transports nutrients, oxygenates your cells and helps in all metabolic processes.

You could observe and think that water is the simplest thing there is. If you look closely at a molecule of water (H_2O), you realize that the percentage of oxygen is eight times greater than hydrogen. The mass percent of the two hydrogen atoms is equal to 11.11%, while the mass percent of an oxygen atom is equal to 88.89%. Over 88% of the water content is oxygen.

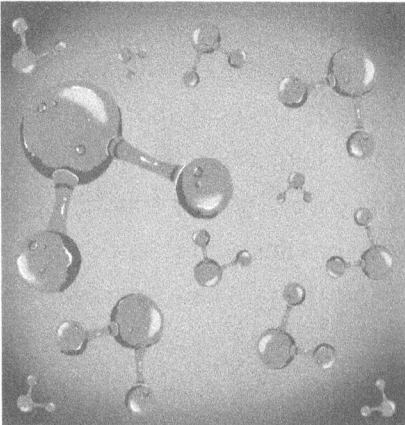

It is really fascinating that when you drink water, you literally drink oxygen. Water gives each cell the ability to breathe and carry out its internal combustion to generate energy[44]. Oxygen creates combustion. There is no combustion without oxygen. Having a slow metabolism means that there is a deficiency in creating energy. If you increase oxygen, you increase the internal combustion of each cell. Something as simple as drinking water is, at the same time, very important.

Why is this not reported to the public? Why are there no commercials or propaganda explaining this? Why not empower lives more with this great truth? I think you already know why. Water does not make as much money as medicine.

Restoring the metabolism is like turning on all the lights in a house that was partially or almost totally dark, because it had too many lights out. You can create energy in dead cells simply by giving your body water.

Listen to your body. Notice when you feel a lot of energy and do not tire easily. This means that you provided your cells with the water and food it needs. Drinking water restores energy to each cell, increasing your metabolism. A healthy metabolism is synonymous with a lot of energy, wanting to move. A slow metabolism feels like your body is crawling, like it's being forced to move, a sign that cells aren't producing energy.

The chemical energy that healthy cells produce is known as Adenosine Triphosphate, or ATP for short. It is what allows movement, what we call life. The main characteristic of life in the body is movement. When your cells make more ATP, you will feel more energy. Without ATP there is no life in your cells, there is no health. A molecule of ATP produces 600 units of energy.

What I find wonderful is that ATP production is much higher in the presence of oxygen. If you combine water with ATP, a chemical reaction occurs, and the energy effect is multiplier: the available energy of ATP increases from 600 units to 6,435 (kilojoules). This is truly fascinating: water activates the metabolism by boosting ATP by a factor of 10^{45}. Water increases the energy (metabolism) of each cell. Oxygen is required during oxidative phosphorylation[46], which is the final stage of cellular respiration.

If oxygen is not present, your cells do not synthesize more ATP. Without enough ATP, cells cannot carry out the reactions they need to function and may even die after a certain period. The next time you drink water, remember that what you drink is oxygen for your cells, which is a life-creating material.

How's Your Habitat?

Have you ever looked closely at a clean fish tank, where you can see every living species with great clarity? You can appreciate incredible and different maritime life when they're in a clean environment. We find the water in that habitat inside and outside of every form of life that inhabits it.

Your body is very similar to a water habitat, where that vital fluid is inside and outside your cells.

Most of the water in your body is within your cells and is known as intracellular fluid. The water inside the cells has dissolved elements, the main one being potassium. The water outside the cells is rich in nutrients and various vital components, where sodium is the dominant element. This fluid is called extracellular water. The extracellular fluid bathes the cells on the outside, but it also circulates in the organs, like plasma, which is an important part of the blood. Also, it is part of the cerebrospinal fluid that circulates between the ventricles of the brain and the spinal cord.

Cell walls regulate both fluids (intracellular and extracellular)[47]: nutrients go in, waste goes out. Let me remind you that the cell membrane is like an envelope and represents its nervous system, because it evaluates the external and internal environment and allows the necessary changes to keep the cell alive.

Your body uses fluids to remove toxins and waste. You need water to detoxify your body. A detoxified body is a healthy body. How is your body's habitat? Is it like a clean fish tank, where the water flows and gives life to each species? Or is the water so cloudy that it is difficult for your habitat to carry out its functions? Your body has the innate ability to cleanse itself of toxins and waste, but it can get to where the pollution of your habitat is too much.

Remember, many times different pains and illnesses are a sign of intoxication in some part of the body. The body warns you; it gives you signs. If you just learn to listen to it, you can consciously heal and make it easier for you to make day-to-day decisions that support your health.

How much water does your body require? It depends on your body. It would be like comparing two houses, one being a small house and the other a huge mansion. The small house requires less water for its functions than the huge mansion. Likewise, in humans, the amount of water required is relative to the size of the body. An easy formula is: divide your weight in pounds by sixteen, and that is the number of eight-ounce glasses a day you should consume[48]. This can vary, for example, if your diet is high in sweets or you smoke, because your body becomes dehydrated, or if you sweat a lot because of the weather or exercise.

Remember, every day is different, and your body has different physiological needs. I suggest you drink water at room temperature, not cold, and definitely not with ice. Your body has an internal temperature that deserves to be respected. That makes it easier for you to carry out your different internal functions.

Drink water during the day, but limit drinking water or any other beverage while eating, since gastric juices get diluted and food is not digested and absorbed optimally. For most, it is a habit to sit down to eat and drink at the same time, but it is not the healthiest for your digestion. Do the test. You will notice the difference after eating. You will not feel so drained of energy, nor so full of gas when you get up from the table. If you consume foods that contain water, such as foods from the land—vegetables, legumes, vegetables—it will be easier for you not to drink when you eat than if you eat a steak with french fries.

The water in our body is not static; it disappears little by little with the different physiological processes[49]. **We lose two to three liters of water daily through our skin when we sweat, breathe, urinate, defecate, and cry.**

If the water content drops by 10%, physiological abnormalities can occur, while a 20% loss of water can devastate your body[50].

For example, some of those physiological changes due to not having enough water in the body can be cardiovascular, as the vasopressin hormone increases[51]. Vasopressin is the hormone that retains fluid, preventing you from urinating, and closes blood vessels to save and prevent water loss. This causes the renin hormone to rise, which raises blood pressure. **Something as basic as drinking water can lower blood pressure.**

The quantity and quality of water in your body also impact your nervous system. Think about your brain for a moment, which controls all processes in the body by sending and receiving electrical signals through the nervous system. As in any communications network, the clarity and speed of the signal depends on the signal-to-noise ratio. If the liquid contains toxic chemicals or metals, the result can be a delay and distortion in the signal, leading to disorders in the nervous system, such as cognitive problems, forgetfulness and mood swings.

Another important fact is that a brain without water contracts and must work harder to achieve the same results as a hydrated brain[52]. In addition, it activates a series of adaptation mechanisms to remain active despite the lack of water. It is vital for your body to replace the necessary water. There is a lot to learn from the water.

I encourage you to look up the book *The Four Phases of Water: Beyond solid, liquid and vapor* written by Gerald H. Pollack, a professor of bioengineering at the University of Washington, Seattle. Pollack devoted himself to studying water in a fascinating way.

Look at nature. Water is the force that moves it. We can learn a lot from it. Every living being hydrates with water, but humans are the only ones who seek to satisfy their thirst with anything other than water. Hydrate yourself with water, the life-creating substance.

Movement Is Life

Every day is a rebirth, a new beginning. Your body always forgives you, even though your habits may not have been the best in the past, and it can heal. Health is normal. Being healthy is your natural state and within yourself, you have all the tools to return to that natural state of health. Recognize that you are gaining skills in a learning process that seeks complete health.

What gift could you give your body that is really meaningful? Exercising your body represents an attribute, a gift. Realize that your body is going to outlast many of the material things you may focus on before you even think about exercising. Many people spend too much time sitting, at work, driving, or at home.

Your body is designed to move.

Having a healthy lifestyle that includes exercise is a personal decision for everyone, but you can certainly inspire others and carry the message to those who seek your help. Remember, your body does what your mind tells it to do. If one of your phrases is "I don't have time to exercise," then it will be so. You won't find the time, because exercising is not a priority for you. Love and value your body enough to have a lifestyle that supports your health. Take a few minutes each day to exercise wisely.

Many follow fashions and trends, and for this reason, they decide to abandon their new exercise routine in a short amount of time. You must know which physical activity is best for you. Find activities you enjoy doing and that make you feel good. There are so many options: walking, dancing, jumping, running, swimming, cycling, yoga, Tai Chi, tennis, golf, whatever you want to do, just start moving your body.

There will always be an activity for everyone, and it doesn't have to be the same every day or for a lifetime. It can change over time, just as you, your environment, your tastes, and your friendships change. Each person is different. Choose consciously.

Start small. The changes you will see in your body, mind, and spirit will amaze you. You want the ability to run, jump, be flexible, and move with ease until the end of your days. **Exercise is vital to maintaining optimal health, keeping your body vigorous, your mind alive, and your spirit free.**

How Does Your Body Benefit From Exercise?

Oxygenation and the Growth Hormone

Two vital organs come into play in oxygenation: the heart and the lungs. Your lungs bring oxygen to the body, providing energy and removing carbon dioxide, the waste product created by producing energy. Your heart sends oxygen to the muscles that are exercising.

During exercise, your body uses more energy and produces more carbon dioxide[53]. To accomplish this, your breathing increases from fifteen times per minute (twelve liters of air) to forty-sixty times per minute (100 liters of air). Your circulation increases to send oxygen to your body and keep your muscles moving.

There are those who love to exercise their body, while others avoid it at all costs. Some of my favorite exercises are short-duration, high-intensity exercises[54]. The quality and intensity of the exercise have more effect than the quantity. It takes twelve to twenty minutes a day and I can do it at home, so time and place are not a problem. We also known them as surge training or HIIT. The key is for your heart rate to increase by 80% - 90%.

Research shows that this type of exercise increases oxygenation and metabolism and stops aging in highly effective ways[55]. One of the greatest benefits of this type of exercise is the increase in the production of growth hormone (GH), which handles several aspects of health such as an increase of energy and endurance, reduction of fat accumulation, an increase of muscle mass, an increase in bone density, an improvement in libido and sexual performance, a reduction in blood pressure, and improvements in sleep patterns and moods.

As I already mentioned, you can choose how to move. Maybe you like walking, swimming, dancing, cycling, using an elliptical machine, full-body movements like squats, and jogging. Do what you like to do, but start moving.

Exercise Reduces Inflammation

Exercise decreases inflammation signals such as interleukin-6 (IL-6) and C-reactive protein (CRP)[56]. This is a great benefit, since inflammation is a large part of the origin and progression of various diseases and disorders of the body and brain. The truth is that exercise has many effects on different organs and systems of the body.

Exercise Keeps You Young

Exercise is linked to more years of life. Studies such as that of A. Tucker in the Preventive Medicine Journal describe how exercise is associated with the length of telomeres, the final part of chromosomes[57]. I emphasize that telomeres are like a shield that protects the DNA of your cells. This final part of the chromosome shortens over the years and with each division of cells, to multiply and regenerate tissues and organs in your body.

People who live longer have telomeres in a more optimal state in relation to others. Your state of consciousness and the decisions you make daily can do a lot to affect the rate at which telomeres shorten. Actually, all the recommendations that I give you from the beginning of this book can help you greatly in this.

Telomere length is measured in base pairs, which are pairs of complementary and opposite nucleotides. There is evidence that people who exercise regularly have telomeres averaging 140 base pairs longer compared to sedentary people. This represents nine years of reduction in cellular aging.

How Does Your Brain Benefit From Exercise?

Exercise Contributes to Neurogenesis

As I mentioned before, in recent years it became clear that the brain can create new neurons, a process known as neurogenesis, and meditation increases neurogenesis. Another factor that favors the growth of new neurons is aerobic exercise[58].

The hippocampus is the area of the brain known to be most capable of growing new cells, and it is a key place for functions like learning and memory. On the other hand, when faced with depression and dementia, it shrinks. It is really important that you recognize that you can create your health with a healthy lifestyle.

Exercise Mitigates and Prevents Depression

Depression is a leading cause of disability throughout the world[59]. Treatments tend to have side effects and are often ineffective. Notably, studies have strongly evidenced that physical activity can mitigate depression[60], while a low level of exercise is a significant risk factor[61].

Physical activity generates serotonin, the happiness hormone, which creates an antidepressant effect. The effect of this hormone is not limited only to the moment of exercise. If you exercise regularly, the concentration of this hormone will grow steadily in your brain. I understand that when a person is depressed, physical activity may be the last thing they want to do, but even a little exercise daily can make a difference.

Exercise Reduces the Risk of Developing Dementia

Studies show that the risk of developing dementia, such as Alzheimer's disease, is significantly reduced when the person exercises[62]. The benefits of exercise are present even if the person begins to exercise when they are older. The brain can grow just like a muscle that gets stronger over time (neuroplasticity). Research tells us that exercise can affect the hippocampus positively, increase sympathetic plasticity, and strengthen nerve impulses[63].

How Does Your Spirit Benefit From Exercise?

I could go on to name more benefits of exercise, but despite knowing the countless benefits that physical activity has on your body, that may not be enough motivation to start a lifestyle that includes physical activity. That motivation has to come from something deeper, not from something external. If your only goal is to lose weight, exercising will most likely feel like punishment for everything you ever ate.

Your body is your house, your temple (1 Corinthians 6:19). Your spirit, your connection to the divine resides in it. Taking care of your body is taking care of your home. Find your reason for exercising.

Three benefits of exercise that I find of great significance in my life are:

Consciousness - When you exercise, it is easier to be more conscious in the present moment. You are more aware of your body and you learn more easily to listen to it.

Intuition - By exercising, you strengthen your heart and its circulation improves, as well as the circulation in the rest of your body. When your blood is flowing better, your mind can be clearer and can hear your heart. Remember that intuition comes from the wisdom of the heart. This helps you to be more connected to yourself.

Creativity - By exercising, you gain greater concentration and strengthen your creativity, since you can look at things from a deeper and healthier point of view. Also, you develop mental flexibility as you make your body more flexible. Creativity is your ability to create new ideas and concepts, and with it, you can find better solutions to your day-to-day circumstances. It is much more than a word; it is an attitude, a way of perceiving life in a useful and original way.

Everything that humans do is essentially an expression of who they are. Leading an active life is an expression. Every good thing you do for yourself is an act of love for yourself, and loving yourself is the foundation for fulfillment in every stage of your life. **Bring life and love to your body by giving it movement.**

LAST LINES...

You are a divine being. You couldn't be more beautiful, powerful, and full of love than you already are. I want you to understand that your life is about discovering who you are and being that entity in its entirety.

Health and plenitude are your right and privilege; they have been since the day you were born.

Keep in mind that being healthy means being complete and whole. It is a state of integrity in all the parts that make you up—your body, mind and spirit. Feeling healthy and whole means being complete in all phases of your life. Being free from disease and illness is only a minimal part of your health. **When you feel like a complete human being, connected with your body, mind and spirit, then you will experience health.**

I hope you feel inspired and motivated to transcend, to live in health and fulfillment in every area of your life. We are together on this journey.

"I alone cannot change the world, but I can throw a rock into the water to generate many waves" - anonymous.

This book represents that rock thrown into the water; if it can generate some beautiful waves of change in you, it will have achieved its purpose.

With you in my heart,

Cesia.

ANNEX:

Tables About Nutrition

Here are several tables with important foods that will help you throughout this learning process. Maybe you are not familiar with some of these foods, and that's normal, because they are not part of your regular diet. My wish in this process is that you can see the great abundance of food that the Earth offers you.

Vegetables

CHARD	BROCCOLINI	SHALLOTS	BELGIAN ESCAROLA	OKRA
CHICORY/RED CHICORY	BAMBOO SHOOS	PARSNIP	ASPARAGUS	HEART OF PALM
ARTICHOKES	SOY SPROUTS/ SOYBEAN GERM	CABBAGE LEAVES	SPINACH	CUCUMBER
CELERY	BOK CHOY	BRUSSELS SPROUTS	FENNEL	PEPPERS
ARUGULA	ZUCCHINI	CAULIFLOWER	BERZA LEAVES	OSTRA PLANTS
SWEET PO-TATO	PUMPKIN	SWEDE	MUSTARD LEAVES	LEEK
EGGPLANT	WATER CHESTNUTS	KALE	TURNKEY LEAVES	RADISH
WATERCRESS	ONION	DANDELION	BEET LEAVES	CABBAGEHEAD
BEET	CHIVES	ENDIVIAS / ESCAROLA	JICAMA	YUCCA
BROCCOLI	MUSHROOMS	GREEN BEANS	TURNIP	CARROT

Fruits

GUAVA	COCONUT	JUJUBES / RED DATE	APPLES	PINEAPPLE
AVOCADO	DATES	CASSAVA	PASSION FRUIT	BANANA / PLANTAIN
APRICOTS	PEACHES	KIWI	MELON	QUENEPA FRUIT
BLUEBERRIES	RASPBERRY	KUMQUATS	BLACK-BERRIES	WATER-MELON
SAUCO FRUIT .	STRAWBERRY	LYCHEE	ORANGE	NASEBERRY
STARFRUIT	POMEGRANATE	LIMES	NECTARINES	TAMARIND
CHERRIES	CURRANT	LEMONS	OLIVES	TOMATO
CUSTARD APPLE	SOURSOP	LOQUATS	PAPAYA	GRAPES
PLUM	GUAVA	MANDARINES	PEAR	
CLEMENTINES	FIGS	MANGO	PERSIMMONS	

Meats and Vegan Proteins

VEGAN	MEAT	FISH
EDAMAME	TURKEY	COD
PEAS	DUCK	HALIBUT
BEANS (BLACK, KIDNEY, WHITE)	CHICKEN	HERRING
CHICKPEAS	LEAN BEEF	MAHI MAHI
SPLIT PEAS	LEAN BUFFALO MEAT	CABALLA
BROAD BEANS	LEAN DEER MEAT	SALMON
BLACK BEANS		SEA BASS
LENTILS		TROUT
NUTS		TUNA
TEMPEH, TOFU		

Good Fats

AVOCADO OIL	AVOCADO
COCONUT OIL	CLARIFIED BUTTER
HIGH OLEIC SUNFLOWER OIL	PEANUTBUTTER
LINSEED OIL	HEMP SEEDS
EXTRA VIRGIN OLIVE OIL	CHIA SEEDS
SESAME SEED OIL	SESAME SEEDS
GRAPESEED OIL	PISTACHIOS

Healthy Grains

AMARANTH

WILD RICE, BASMATI, WHOLE WHEAT

WHOLE OATS

BARLEY

QUINOA

TEFF

BUCKWHEAT GROATS

Spices

GARLIC	CHILI POWDER	DILL	MUSTARD	ROSEMARY
BASIL	CILANTRO	TARRAGON	NUTMEG	SEA SALT
ANNIS	CLOVES	VANILLA EXTRACT	OREGANO	SAGE
SAFFRON	CUMIN	LEMONGRASS	PARSLEY	THYME
CINNAMON	TURMERIC	BAYLEAVES	CAYENNE PEPPER	
CARDAMOM	CURRY	GINGER	BLACK PEPPER	
CHIVES	JUNIPER	MINT	PAPRIKA	

Seeds

POPPY

HEMP

CHIA

PUMPKIN

SUNFLOWER

FLAX

SESAME

Sugars

COCONUT SUGAR

DATE SUGAR

MONK FRUIT SUGAR

BANANAS

DATES

STEVIA - WHOLE LEAF (POWDER OR LIQUID)

Vinegars

BALSAMIC VINEGAR

APPLE CIDER VINEGAR

SHERRY VINEGAR

WHITE WINE VINEGAR

RED WINE VINEGAR

Foods That Support the Liver

VITAMINS, MINERALS, ENZYMES. ANTIOXIDANTS	BROCCOLI, RADISH, LEEKS, SPINACH, ONIONS, GARLIC, CELERY, CABBAGE, BRUSSELS SPANISH, EDAMAME, WALNUTS, GRAPEFRUIT, LEMON, CARROT, GREEN APPLE, SPINACH, GREEN TEA, PUMPKIN SEED
CINARINE	ARTICHOKES, THISTLE, GINGER, LEMON, TURMERIC, APPLE, CUCUMBER, BETABEL (BEETROOT), CELERY, PARSLEY
GLUTATHIONE	SPINACH, WATERMELON, ASPARAGUS, AVOCADO, PUMPKIN, TOMATOES, CRUCIFEROUS VEGETABLES (RUGULA OR ARUGULA, BROCCOLI, CABBAGE, BRUSSELS, CAULIFLOWER, GREEN LEAF VEGETABLES), WALNUTS, GARLIC
VITAMIN C	GRAPE, LEMON
VITAMIN E	WALNUTS, SEEDS, GREEN LEAF VEGETABLES (SPINACH, BROCCOLI) AVOCADO
AMINOACIDS	HEMP SEEDS, NUTS, PISTACHIOS, LEGUMES LIKE CHICKPEAS, QUINOA, AMARANTH
VITAMIN B	WHOLE CEREALS, OATS, QUINOA, BEANS, CHICKPEAS, BEANS, BEANS

Author's Profile

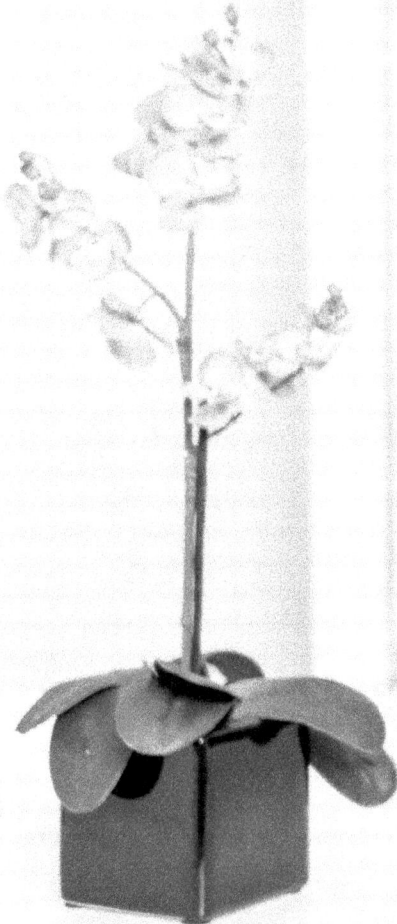

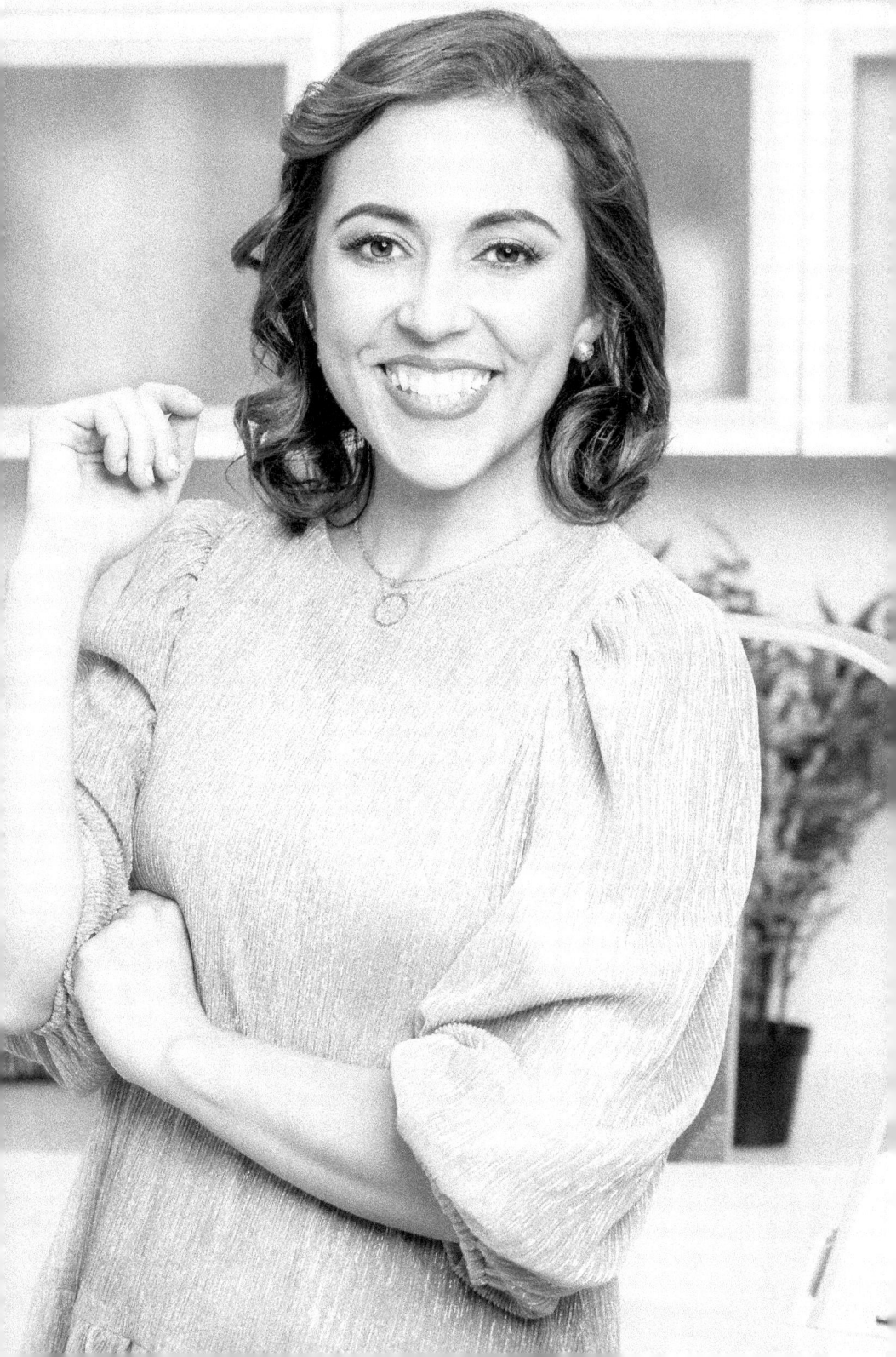

Dr. Cesia Estebané is a renowned chiropractor and health and wellness expert, graduated from *Cleveland University - Kansas City* in 2009. She has dedicated her life to carrying out her mission: to help thousands of people heal their lives and bodies inside out.

Born in the country of Mexico, she is the mother of two children and her best friend's wife. She currently lives and enjoys a successful chiropractic practice in Puerto Rico, where she has been practicing for over eleven years alongside her colleague and husband.

As an educator, her main motivation is the conviction that each person has the potential for full health and abundance in every area of their life.

Besides offering classes online, she teaches live workshops where she uses her knowledge to help others heal physically, emotionally, and spiritually. Her teaching style is inspiring, easy to understand, and compassionate. Since she was a child, her love and passion for people distinguish her, and motivates her to be a faithful practitioner and researcher of the human potential.

Bibliography

1. Oleribe, O. O., Ukwedeh, O., Burstow, N. J., Gomaa, A. I., Sonderup, M. W., Cook, N., Waked, I., Spearman, W., & Taylor-Robinson, S. D. (2018). Health: redefined. The Pan African medical journal, 30, 292. https://doi.org/10.11604/pamj.2018.30.292.15436.

2. Peruzzotti-Jametti, L., Donegá, M., Giusto, E., Mallucci, G., Marchetti, B., & Pluchino, S. (2014). The role of the immune system in central nervous system plasticity after acute injury. Neuroscience, 283, 210–221. https://doi.org/10.1016/j.neuroscience.2014.04.036

3. Neil Z. Miller (2016). Millers Review of Critical Vaccine Studies: 400 Important Scientific Papers Summarized for Parents and Researchers.

4. Mason, J. W., Ramseth, D. J., Chanter, D. O., Moon, T. E., Goodman, D. B., Mendzelevski, B. (2017). Electrocardiographic reference ranges derived from 79,743 ambulatory subjects. Journal of Electrocardiology, 40-3, 228-234. Retrieved from https://doi.org/10.1016/j.jelectrocard.2006.09.003

5. Boxym. (2019) How Much Oxygen Does a Person Consume in a Day. Retrieved from https://boxym.com/how-much-oxygen-does-a-person-consume-in-a-day/

6. Institute for Quality and Efficiency in Health Care (IQWiG). (2009). How does the stomach work? InformedHealth.org [Internet]. Retrieved from https://www.ncbi.nlm.nih.gov/books/NBK279304/

7. Society for Neuroscience. Brain Awareness Campaign. Retrieved from https://www.sfn.org/BAW

8. Harvard-Smithsonian Center for Astrophysics. NASA's Chandra X-ray Observatory. Retrieved from https://chandra.harvard.edu/about/

9. Lipton, B. (2005). The Biology of Belief: Unleashing the Power of Consciousness, Matter & Miracles. P. 84.

10. Lipton, B. (2005). The Biology of Belief: Unleashing the Power of Consciousness, Matter & Miracles. P. 109.

11. Lipton, B. (2005). The Biology of Belief: Unleashing the Power of Consciousness, Matter & Miracles. P. 87, 98.

12. Glorioso, J., Jacoby, J. (2005). An interview with David Baltimore. Gene Therapy Journal. Retrieved from https://doi.org/10.1038/sj.gt.3302526

13. Lipton, B. (2005). The Biology of Belief: Unleashing the Power of Consciousness, Matter & Miracles. P. 87-88.

14. Hay, L. (1990). Heart Thoughts: A Treasury of Inner Wisdom. P. 118.

15. Gustafson C. (2017). Bruce Lipton, PhD: The Jump From Cell Culture to Consciousness. Integrative medicine (Encinitas, Calif.), 16(6), 44-50.

16. Gustafson C. (2017). Bruce Lipton, PhD: The Jump From Cell Culture to Consciousness. Integrative medicine (Encinitas, Calif.), 16(6), 44-50.

17. McCraty, Rollin & Mike, Atkinson & Tomasino, Dana & Bradley, Raymond. (2009). The Coherent Heart Heart-Brain Interactions, Psychophysiological Coherence, and the Emergence of System-Wide Order. Integral Review. P. 41.

18. McCraty, Rollin. (2016). Science of the Heart, Volume 2 Exploring the Role of the Heart in Human Performance An Overview of Research Conducted by the HeartMath Institute. 10.13140/RG.2.1.3873.5128.

19. McCraty, R., & Zayas, M. A. (2014). Cardiac coherence, self-regulation, autonomic stability, and psychosocial well-being. Frontiers in psychology, 5, 1090. Retrieved from https://doi.org/10.3389/fpsyg.2014.01090

20. McCraty, R., Atkinson, P. D. M., & Tomasino, D. (2003). Modulation of DNA conformation by heart-focused intention. HeartMath Research Center, Institute of HeartMath, Publication (03-008), 2.

21. McCraty, R., Atkinson, P. D. M., & Tomasino, D. (2003). Modulation of DNA conformation by heart-focused intention. HeartMath Research Center, Institute of HeartMath, Publication (03-008), 2.

22. McCraty, R., Atkinson, P. D. M., & Tomasino, D. (2003). Modulation of DNA conformation by heart-focused intention. HeartMath Research Center, Institute of HeartMath, Publication (03-008), 2.

23. Braden, G. Human by Design. The Shift Network Online Course. Module 1.

24. Holthaus, G. (2008), Learning Native Wisdom: What Traditional Cultures Teach Us About Subsistence, Sustainibility, and Spirtuality. University Press of Kentucky. P. 170.

25. Hodges, R. E., & Minich, D. M. (2015). Modulation of Metabolic Detoxification Pathways Using Foods and Food-Derived Components: A Scientific Review with Clinical Application. Journal of nutrition and metabolism, 2015, 760689. Retrieved from https://doi.org/10.1155/2015/760689

26. Grube, A., Donaldson, D., Kiely, T., Wu, L.(2011). Pesticides Industry Sales and Usage 2006 and 2007 Market Estimates. U.S. Environmental Protection Agency. Retrieved from http://www.epa.gov/sites/production/files/2015-10/documents/market_estimates2007.pdf.

27. Thornton, J. W., McCaly, M., Houlihan, J. (2002). Biomonitoring of Industrial Pollutants: Health and Policy Implications of the Chemical Body Burden. Public Health Reports 117(4): 315-23.

28. National Toxicology Program. Annual Report for Fiscal Year 2018. U.S. Department of Health and Human Services. Retrieved from https://ntp.niehs.nih.gov/annualreport/2018/2018annualreportdownloadpdf.pdf

29. O'Reilly, G. A., Belcher, B. R., Davis, J. N., Martinez, L. T., Huh, J., Antunez-Castillo, L., Weigensberg, M., Goran, M. I., & Spruijt-Metz, D. (2015). Effects of high-sugar and high-fiber meals on physical activity behaviors in Latino and African American adolescents. Obesity (Silver Spring, Md.), 23(9), 1886–1894. https://doi.org/10.1002/oby.21169

30. Orgel, E., & Mittelman, S. D. (2013). The links between insulin resistance, diabetes, and cancer. Current diabetes reports, 13(2), 213–222. https://doi.org/10.1007/s11892-012-0356-6

31. Tasevska, N., Jiao, L., Cross, A. J., Kipnis, V., Subar, A. F., Hollenbeck, A., Schatzkin, A., & Potischman, N. (2012). Sugars in diet and risk of cancer in the NIH-AARP Diet and Health Study. International journal of cancer, 130(1), 159–169. https://doi.org/10.1002/ijc.25990

32. Guo, X., Park, Y., Freedman, N. D., Sinha, R., Hollenbeck, A. R., Blair, A., & Chen, H. (2014). Sweetened beverages, coffee, and tea and depression risk among older US adults. PloS one, 9(4), e94715. https://doi.org/10.1371/journal.pone.0094715

33. Akbaraly, T. N., Brunner, E. J., Ferrie, J. E., Marmot, M. G., Kivimaki, M., & Singh-Manoux, A. (2009). Dietary pattern and depressive symptoms in middle age. The British journal of psychiatry : the journal of mental science, 195(5), 408–413. https://doi.org/10.1192/bjp.bp.108.058925

34. Lee, D., Hwang, W., Artan, M., Jeong, D. E., & Lee, S. J. (2015). Effects of nutritional components on aging. Aging cell, 14(1), 8–16. https://doi.org/10.1111/acel.12277

35. Casares, D., Escribá, P. V., & Rosselló, C. A. (2019). Membrane Lipid Composition: Effect on Membrane and Organelle Structure, Function and Compartmentalization and Therapeutic Avenues. International journal of molecular sciences, 20(9), 2167. Retrieved from https://doi.org/10.3390/ijms20092167

36. U.S. Food & Drug. (2018). Final Determination Regarding Partially Hydrogenated Oils (Removing Trans Fat). Retrieved from https://www.fda.gov/food/food-additives-petitions/final-determination-regarding-partially-hydrogenated-oils-removing-trans-fat

37. Takeuchi, H., Sugano, M. (2017). Industrial Trans Fatty Acid and Serum Cholesterol: The Allowable Dietary Level. Journal of Lipids. 1-10.

38. Hall, K., Ayuketah, A., Brychta, R., Cai, H., Cassimatis, T., Chen, K. Y., Chung, S. T., Costa, E., Courville, A., Darcey, V., Fletcher, L. A., Forde, C. G., Gharib, A. M., Guo, J., Howard, R., Joseph, P. V., McGhee, S., Ouwerkerk, R., Raisinger, K., Rozga, I., Stagliano, M., Walter, M., Walter, P. J., Yand, S., Zhou, M. (2019). Ultra-Processed Diets Cause Excess Calorie Intake and Weight Gain: An Inpatient Randomized Controlled Trial of Ad Libitum Food Intake. Cell Metabolism. 30(1).

39. Jéquier, E., Constant, F. (2010). Water as an essential nutrient: the physiological basis of hydration. European Journal of Clinical Nutrition. 64, 115–123. Retrieved from https://doi.org/10.1038/ejcn.2009.111

40. O'Brien JS, Sampson EL. (1965). Lipid composition of the normal human brain: gray matter, white matter, and myelin. Journal of Lipid Research. V6.

41. Mitchell, H. H., Hamilton, T. S., Steggerda F. R., Bean, H. W., (1945). The Chemical Composition of the Adult Human Body and its Bearing on the Biochemistry of Growth. University of Illinois. Retrieved from https://www.jbc.org/content/158/3/625.full.pdf

42. The Franklin Institute Inc. Your Living Blood: It's Alive! - What's it made of? Retrieved from https://www.fi.edu/heart/its-alive

43. Water Science School. The Water in You: Water and the Human Body. U.S. Geological Survey. Retrieved from https://www.usgs.gov/special-topic/water-science-school/science/water-you-water-and-human-body?qt-science_center_objects=0#qt-science_center_objects

44. Lorenzo, I., Serra-Prat, M., & Yébenes, J. C. (2019). The Role of Water Homeostasis in Muscle Function and Frailty: A Review. Nutrients, 11(8), 1857. https://doi.org/10.3390/nu11081857

45. Suarez, F., (2009) Diabetes Sin Problemas: EL Control de la Diabetes con la Ayuda del Poder del Metabolismo.

46. Hroudová, J., & Fišar, Z. (2013). Control mechanisms in mitochondrial oxidative phosphorylation. Neural regeneration research, 8(4), 363-375. https://doi.org/10.3969/j.issn.1673-5374.2013.04.009

47. Jéquier, E., Constant, F. (2010). Water as an essential nutrient: the physiological basis of hydration. European Journal of Clinical Nutrition 64, 115-123. https://doi.org/10.1038/ejcn.2009.111

48. Batmanghelidj, F. (1997). The Body's Many Cries for Water.

49. Szinnai, G., Schachinger, H., Arnaud, M. J., Linder, L., Keller, U. (2005). Water and Electrolyte Homeostasis: Effect Of Water Deprivation On Cognitive-Motor Performance In Healthy Men And Women. American Journal of Physiology-Regulatory, Integrative and Comparative Physiology. 289 (1). Retrieved from https://journals.physiology.org/doi/full/10.1152/ajpregu.00501.2004

50. Jang S, Cheon C, Jang BH, Park S, Oh SM, Shin YC, Ko SG. (2016). Relationship Between Water Intake and Metabolic/Heart Diseases: Based on Korean National Health and Nutrition Examination Survey (KNHANES). Osong Public Health and Research Perspective. 7(5):289-295. doi:10.1016/j.phrp.2016.08.007.

51. Watso JC, Farquhar WB. (2019). Hydration Status and Cardiovascular Function. Nutrients. 11(8):1866. doi: 10.3390/nu11081866.

52. Ritz, P., & Berrut, G. (2005). The importance of good hydration for day-to-day health. Nutrition reviews, 63(6 Pt 2), S6–S13. https://doi.org/10.1111/j.1753-4887.2005.tb00155.x

53. Your lungs and exercise. (2016). Breathe (Sheffield, England), 12(1), 97–100. https://doi.org/10.1183/20734735.ELF121

54. Robinson, M. M., Dasari, S., Konopka, A. R., Johnson, M. L., Manjunatha, S., Esponda, R. R., Carter, R. E., Lanza, I. R., & Nair, K. S. (2017). Enhanced Protein Translation Underlies Improved Metabolic and Physical Adaptations to Different Exercise Training Modes in Young and Old Humans. Cell metabolism, 25(3), 581–592. https://doi.org/10.1016/j.cmet.2017.02.009

55. Boutcher S. H. (2011). High-intensity intermittent exercise and fat loss. Journal of obesity, 2011, 868305. https://doi.org/10.1155/2011/868305

56. Dimitrov, S., Hulteng, E., & Hong, S. (2017). Inflammation and exercise: Inhibition of monocytic intracellular TNF production by acute exercise via 2-adrenergic activation. Brain, behavior, and immunity, 61, 60–68. https://doi.org/10.1016/j.bbi.2016.12.017

57. Tucker L. A. (2017). Physical activity and telomere length in U.S. men and women: An NHANES investigation. Preventive medicine, 100, 145-151. https://doi.org/10.1016/j.ypmed.2017.04.027

58. Nokia, M. S., Lensu, S., Ahtiainen, J. P., Johansson, P. P., Koch, L. G., Britton, S. L., & Kainulainen, H. (2016). Physical exercise increases adult hippocampal neurogenesis in male rats provided it is aerobic and sustained. The Journal of physiology, 594(7), 1855-1873. https://doi.org/10.1113/JP271552

59. News Release. (2019). "Depression: let's talk" says WHO, as depression tops list of causes of ill health. World Health Organization. Retrieved from https://www.who.int/news/item/30-03-2017--depression-let-s-talk-says-who-as-depression-tops-list-of-causes-of-ill-health#:~:text=WHO-,%22Depression%3A%20let's%20talk%22%20says%20WHO%2C%20as%20depression%20tops,of%20causes%20of%20ill%20health&text=Depression%20is%20the%20leading%20cause,18%25%20between%202005%20and%202015.

60. Hearing, C. M., Chang, W. C., Szuhany, K. L., Deckersbach, T., Nierenberg, A. A., & Sylvia, L. G. (2016). Physical Exercise for Treatment of Mood Disorders: A Critical Review. Current behavioral neuroscience reports, 3(4), 350-359. https://doi.org/10.1007/s40473-016-0089-y

61. Holmquist, S., Mattsson, S., Schele, I., Nordström, P., & Nordström, A. (2017). Low physical activity as a key differentiating factor in the potential high-risk profile for depressive symptoms in older adults. Depression and anxiety, 34(9), 817-825. https://doi.org/10.1002/da.22638

62. Erickson, K. I., Voss, M. W., Prakash, R. S., Basak, C., Szabo, A., Chaddock, L., Kim, J. S., Heo, S., Alves, H., White, S. M., Wojcicki, T. R., Mailey, E., Vieira, V. J., Martin, S. A., Pence, B. D., Woods, J. A., McAuley, E., & Kramer, A. F. (2011). Exercise training increases size of hippocampus and improves memory. Proceedings of the National Academy of Sciences of the United States of America, 108(7), 3017-3022. https://doi.org/10.1073/pnas.1015950108

63. Ellingson, L. D., Meyer, J. D., Shook, R. P., Dixon, P. M., Hand, G. A., Wirth, M. D., Paluch, A. E., Burgess, S., Hebert, J. R., & Blair, S. N. (2018). Changes in sedentary time are associated with changes in mental wellbeing over 1 year in young adults. Preventive medicine reports, 11, 274-281. https://doi.org/10.1016/j.pmedr.2018.07.013

www.ingramcontent.com/pod-product-compliance
Lightning Source LLC
Chambersburg PA
CBHW070248290326
41930CB00042B/2846